NUT JOB

How I Crushed My Food Allergies to Thrive

SONIA HUNT

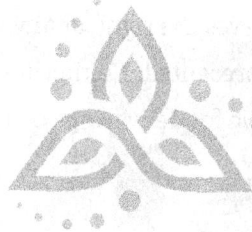

*For my parents, Nita and Vinay, for being on this journey
with me, and encouraging me to evolve in my own beautiful way.*

For Snoop, the little Angel who watches over me.

TABLE OF CONTENTS

INTRODUCTION

I've almost died four times in my life. Nothing heart-stopping like a heart attack, nor psychotic like being shot. Not even bone-crushing like being hit by a car. Each time, the cause of my near death was the juiciest culprit of them all: food.

I am one of over 32 million Americans[1] with severe food allergies. I was first diagnosed with a peanut and tree nut allergy in the late 1970s around the age of three. The icing on my nut-free cake was that I was also diagnosed with severe environmental allergies, and the cherry on top was an asthma diagnosis. The triple threat I always wanted was to be smart, beautiful, and rich, not this whack.

My immigrant parents hailed from India and had never heard the words "food allergy" before. "How could somebody be allergic to food?" they would ask my doctors in their cute Indian accents. "Food is supposed to nourish our bodies, not be deadly." With my diagnosis, I became the broken child amongst siblings who did not share my health issues. Lucky me! As a child, I was constantly in and out of the hospital, either because of food-allergy reactions, asthma-related incidents, or the severe nosebleeds that were a byproduct of my environmental allergies and a bad habit of picking my nose. My childhood was supposed to be all about playing in a sandbox with friends, not about being allergic to the sand itself!

A team of medical professionals became my family's best friends, as we'd see them often to treat my various ailments. My recommended treatment options were a slew of Western prescription medications, immunotherapy in the form of desensitizing allergy shots, and a list of over-the-counter medications—all with harsh side effects. As a family, we were at the mercy of the medical team and the treatment options they recommended seeing as we didn't really know much about my triple diagnosis. Nor did my parents know anyone with food allergies, and in the 1970s, there was no Internet and no WebMD.com to research a diagnosis. There wasn't even a *Dr. Oz Show* kind of television segment about food allergies, so we followed the lead of my doctors. I became what felt like a poster child for allergies and asthma.

Each one of my health diagnoses was related to the other. For example, some airborne substances can trigger allergy or asthma symptoms, and data from the *Journal of Environmental and Public Health* shows that "...an increased urbanization (in the United States) contributes to the environment-food allergy nexus".[2] Environmental allergies are an immune response to something in a person's surroundings that's typically otherwise harmless. Well, *my* list of environmental allergies at the time included dust mites, pollen, trees, mold, and cigarette smoke—all things I was subjected to in the city of Philadelphia, where I grew up. Asthma (which is closely linked to severe reactions to food allergies) is an inflammatory condition of the airways that affects breathing. According to the Asthma and Allergy Foundation of America, "For some people, there may be an indirect connection between food and asthma. Food is not a common asthma trigger. But asthma can be affected by eating. Asthma can also affect how you react if you have food allergies".[3] So, my triple threat became three times as hard to manage.

You're probably thinking, "Damn, this girl is a mess!" You would be correct. And I won't lie—for years, I was the sole guest at my own ultimate and most awesome pity party. It was fun while it lasted and allowed me to wallow in my misery. But once the party was over, I emerged feeling like a loser, which is how I proceeded to see myself for decades because of my health issues. Yet on the outside, I still projected a happy-go-lucky soul.

In my lifetime, I've been to the emergency room 18 times due to my food allergies and four times in a full anaphylaxis condition: twice during childhood, once in college, and the last time in 2008. Those numbers don't include the numerous other visits to the emergency room due to severe nosebleeds and other issues related to my environmental allergies and asthma. My allergic reactions have varied from situation to situation and have included swelling of my lips, tongue, and throat; hives; itchy skin; stomach pain; and shortness of breath. When my stomach hurt or my throat was itching, it was easy to grin and bear it. But the minute I started looking like Will Smith in *Hitch*, I was out the door.

As the wonderful humans they are, my mom and dad pushed my doctors to understand why this was happening and how we could get rid of it quickly and for good. In the 1970s, there was little data on the causes of food allergies, and that situation has not changed much today. However, some hypotheses have emerged over the past ten or so years. For instance, according to a 2016 report by the American College of Allergy, Asthma, and Immunology, "...factors such as race, ethnicity, and genetics contribute to allergy development".[4] Also, research from the National Center for Biotechnology Information shows that "Factors such as hygiene and lack of exposure to microbial factors, composition of the intestinal microbiota, diet, obesity, Vitamin D, and environmental chemical exposure may have contributed to the alarming rise in the rate of food allergies in countries with a Westernized lifestyle".[5] These are only theories, but researchers are working to collect more data to prove these new hypotheses.

The two main things my parents learned about my food allergies back in the 1970s still held true in 2020:

1. There is **no cure** for food allergies.
2. The only way to prevent a reaction is by **not eating the food.**

Countless people around the world are undiagnosed or self-diagnosed with food allergies. I know many of these people! "While we found that 1 in 10 adults have a food allergy, nearly twice as many adults think that they are allergic to foods while their symptoms may suggest food intolerance or other food-related conditions," says Dr. Ruchi Gupta, M.D., MPH, from Lurie Children's Hospital. She is also a professor of pediatrics at the Northwestern University Feinberg School of Medicine.[6]

FARE, the Food Allergy Research & Education organization, reports:[7]

- Every three minutes, a food allergy reaction sends someone to the emergency room.

- Each year in the United States, 200,000 people require emergency medical care for allergic reactions to food.

- About 40% of children with food allergies are allergic to more than one food.

- About 40% of children with food allergies have experienced a severe allergic reaction such as anaphylaxis.

- Studies published in 2018 and 2019 estimated that the following number of Americans of all ages have convincing symptoms of allergy to the following foods:

  - *Shellfish: 8.2 million*

  - *Milk: 6.1 million*

  - *Peanuts: 6.1 million*

  - *Tree nuts: 3.9 million*

  - *Eggs: 2.6 million*

  - *Finfish: 2.6 million*

  - *Wheat: 2.4 million*

- *Soy: 1.9 million*

- *Sesame: 0.7 million*

- Although allergies to milk, egg, wheat, and soy often resolve in childhood, children appear to be outgrowing some of these allergies more slowly than in previous decades, with many children still allergic beyond age five.

- Allergies to peanuts, tree nuts, finfish, and shellfish are generally lifelong.

In addition to this data, millions of people in the world have food sensitivities or intolerances. The difference between a food allergy and a food sensitivity is the body's response: with food *allergies*, the immune system causes the reaction; with food *sensitivities*, the reaction is triggered by the digestive system. This can lead to symptoms such as intestinal gas, abdominal pain, or diarrhea. The "net net," as I like to say, is that today it is almost abnormal to *not* have some form of a food restriction. Data also shows that living in the United States for over ten years may raise the risk of some allergies.[8] Now, that is definitely food for thought!

So, why can't we get our acts together and figure this out? In 1988, Dr. Patricia Bath invented and patented the Laserphaco Probe, which improved treatment for cataract patients. In the 1990s, the Human Genome Project mapped the physical genes that make up the human body. In 1998, the FDA approved the use of Viagra. ('Nuff said.) In the early 2000s, stem cell research was just as hot of a topic as HIV cocktails were. In the late 2010s, countless smoke-free laws were passed, HPV vaccines were introduced, and bionic limbs surfaced. And in 2020, several pharmaceutical companies created a COVID-19 vaccine that rapidly went through an Emergency Use process with the FDA. Yet despite the growth rate of food allergies in the US, doctors still don't know the exact cause of food allergies and we still don't have a cure for them. WTF?

I have often wondered if anyone really cares. Are the over 32 million Americans who suffer not enough? Allergic disease is one of the most common chronic health conditions in the world and is usually considered a disability under the Americans with Disabilities Act.[9]

The number of people with food allergies in the United States continues to rise as time goes on. The Centers for Disease Control and Prevention (CDC) reports that "The prevalence of food allergies in children increased by 50% between 1997 and 2011".[10] In 2017, CBS News reported that "...approximately four percent of Americans have a food allergy, with women and Asians the most affected".[11] Uh, hello...I fall into both of those categories! As data has continued to be released over the decades, the alarming rates of food allergies and incidents are often depressing. But I was stuck in my own hell just having to figure out how to survive.

We've all read too many stories of a child who eats a piece of food, has an immediate reaction to that food, and doesn't survive. It is unfathomable, unacceptable, and unconscionable that we still don't have a handle on food allergies in America.

IT'S TIME TO WAKE UP TO THE FACT THAT FOOD IN THE UNITED STATES IS KILLING US.

YEARS OF HIDING MY ALLERGIES

My parents were always a bit overcautious with me as they'd seen firsthand what happened when a normal meal turned into an instantaneous allergy reaction and a trip to the emergency room. But as a tween who wanted to be independent, it was not fun to have parents gawking, telling me what to eat and what not to eat, and speaking for me when I kinda sorta wanted to speak up for myself. In my tween years, I was also being hit with other issues that I somehow had to reconcile. Those ranged from being one of the only families of color in an all-white Jewish neighborhood to the East-versus-West cultural differences of being Indian versus a first-generation American. I was an impressionable, young brown girl who was scouring magazines like *Seventeen, Glamour,* and *Vogue*—all of which promoted the 5'8," blonde-haired, blue-eyed waif frame as "normal." I looked nothing like that and again felt like a reject. Most of the time, life felt like it was too much for me, but I didn't want to share that feeling with anyone out of shame. I only figured out that that feeling *was* shame years later! So, I kept it all inside, suppressing my life issues just like my medications suppressed my food allergies, and I kept smiling on the outside.

In my full-blown teenage years, I chose to blend in and not draw attention to my food allergies. Throughout my young adulthood, in fact, I continued to suppress my voice to keep up the illusion that I was normal. Incidents would occur, but I would hide them or keep them to myself and my parents. Then in my adult life, something happened that forced me to stop my madness—a single incident finally compelled me to begin taking responsibility and advocating for myself. This turning point came in the year 2008, three decades after I had first been diagnosed with food allergies.

In 2008, there was so much going on in America, including the collapse of the housing bubble that led to the late-2000s recession and the election of the country's first African-American president, a charismatic human by the name of Barack Obama. Historical shifts were upon us as a nation and were about to be upon me as well.

Despite the state of global flux, I began the year 2008 on cloud nine. I was living in San Francisco, California, a place I had moved to ten years prior after having graduated from college. I took advantage of the housing crisis to close on a new home. I had a stable director-level job at a consumer technology company in San Francisco and actually had some savings left after the home purchase. More importantly, I was surrounded by an incredible set of friends who unconditionally supported me in everything I set my mind to do. Seeing that California's lifestyle embeds all things health into your soul, in early 2008 I ran my fourth marathon in Maui, Hawaii, to prove to myself that my-thirty-something body still had it going on.

After the race was over, I spent an extra week lying on the beach in Maui to peace out and write in my journal, thinking about where I wanted to take my career and life. I was at a bit of a crossroads at work, so sleeping on the beach, eating Hawaiian poke, and drinking a Blue Hawaiian while journaling sounded like a perfect way to recover from running 26.2 miles.

The tech culture in San Francisco at the time was all about "Do more, be more!" as if who you were wasn't good enough. At the beginning of my career in Silicon Valley, a peer told me that the ultimate goal for survival in the Valley was to work like a dog in order to climb the corporate ladder, go through an IPO with your company, have a side gig that made extra income, buy a house, find a husband, and make a shit ton of money—all before you turned thirty. It was the tech culture at the time, and we gobbled it up. Can you see a theme of toxicity in my life?

I was feverishly journaling a long list of questions that would help me determine what direction I wanted to head next in my career. At the time, I was working for yet another technology company with a "bro-like" environment that did not take the few women who worked there seriously. It was a miserable place. I didn't realize how unhealthy that work situation was and the effect it was having on me until I started writing in my journal. I wrote down questions like "What am I good at?" and "What areas do I want to grow in?" and "What do I like doing in my work life and in my play life?" and "What do I *not* like to do?" and "Which areas excite me and which don't?" to name a few. It was cathartic to write all of that down and begin to unravel all of the questions running around in my brain. During that one week on the beach, I decided that I was going to leave my current employer and create a new venture that would allow me to tap into the right side of my brain.

Upon returning from the marathon, I spent all of my free time strategizing about what creative venture I could work on. I kept ending up in the food and wine sector as an area of interest. I didn't know *what* I would do in that sector, but it interested me on many levels that were—ironically—also tied to my illness. I was excited and scared about this newfound energy I felt to create something that hopefully would take me in a new, toxicity-free direction in my career and in life!

From a health perspective, in 2008, my body was in great shape (as I had just proved by running another marathon), and it had also been 13 years since I had had any emergent food allergy incidents. What a blessing! I didn't know if it was luck or I had become a rockstar at managing my allergies and asthma on my own. It felt like a little of both. During those 13 years, I did have some itchy, small hives and even some stomach upset, but nothing major that caused me to run to the hospital. I nicknamed those years the "Lucky 13," as everything seemed to be going well post-college and up to that point of my independent life in California.

And then, just like Murphy's Law says, it happened: the Lucky 13 came to an end in the blink of an eye.

Late one night after I had returned from a two-week business trip to China and Hong Kong, I found myself lying on an emergency room table almost dead due to having the worst anaphylactic reaction of my life. That incident changed my existence forever. The diagnosis handed to me was like a hard, back-handed slap across the face: severe allergic reaction to a food substance had caused an onset of anaphylaxis. Wait, *what*? A food allergy? You're kidding. *How*? *Why*?

When I heard the diagnosis from the emergency room doctor, I tried to laugh, but it hurt my lungs too much. I said to the doctor, "Food allergy? Oh no, no. You must be mistaken—I haven't had any food allergy incidents for 13 years! You're wrong."

Still, I knew the situation was bad when I looked down at my arms, which were covered in hives despite the fact that I was hooked up to IVs. My doctor, not amused by my reaction, proceeded to tell me all the gory details of exactly how bad my situation was. She kept me in the emergency room for days before she even considered releasing me.

Why was this happening again? Hadn't the first three anaphylactic incidents in my life been bad enough? This allergic reaction was the worst I had ever had in my entire life, and I had a bad feeling that something else—something even worse—was coming. My body was sick, and now my soul was also sick as I started to question if I had done something wrong that had caused this reaction. Was I managing my food allergies incorrectly? Had I forgotten to tell the restaurant staff something important during dinner? How could I be so healthy for 13 years and all of the sudden be sick again? A voice snuck into my head, saying, "Maybe you only *think* you've been healthy..." This creepy thought came into my brain like a conversation between an angel and the devil.

Before the incident, I had been on top of the world, excited to build a new venture. Now I was almost dead in the emergency room. Maybe this was the Universe's way of trying to teach me a lesson. Because after this fourth time in my life in a full anaphylaxis situation, I just didn't feel like I'd survive another one. And as a parting gift, the Universe gave me one constant reminder of that night, one that led to the lowest point in my life:

I SPENT THE ENTIRE NEXT YEAR COVERED IN HIVES.

Author and podcaster Tim Ferris[12] believes that it's hard to achieve anything meaningful without having some clear direction or results in mind. Up until 2008, I was coasting along in life, with no defined purpose or knowledge of where I was headed because I just didn't look at life that way. But when I was spared yet again by the Universe, it became urgent that I define my mission statement or North Star. I needed to have a fixed destination that I could depend on in life as the world changed around me. I needed a beacon and a navigational tool, something inspiring that I felt connected to in my soul.

The point of having this was to help me make informed daily decisions, allowing me to be happy with my progress and continue to move toward achieving that North Star. Psychologist and *New York Times* best-selling author Rick Hanson states, "What's the light that will guide you out of your own tangled woods—both the woods 'out there' in the world and the ones 'in here,' inside your own mind?"[13] This spoke volumes to me and was exactly what I needed to figure out.

To stay true to my nerdy, techie ways, I went about finding my own North Star by researching other people's Stars. I asked anyone

I met if they had one. I even researched online to see if anyone was writing about their North Star. Most of my friends didn't have a personal North Star written down in a statement, and some felt it was a good exercise to go through alongside me. My online research took me to a person who had a lifelong dream of becoming a surgeon and someone else who wanted to climb Machu Picchu. Interestingly, another kindred spirit was Dr. Govindappa Venkataswamy, an ophthalmologist with crippled fingers who started the Aravind Eye Care System in 1976. Each person's North Star was unique and personal in its own right. There was no right or wrong answer—it just needed to be something that spoke to me. I finally sat peacefully one day and wrote down these words:

My North Star: To age healthily by ridding myself of my food allergies.

The year following my 2008 incident became the most imperative and poignant year in my entire life and would serve as the foundation for years to come. Since I was at rock bottom dealing with hives all over my body for a year, I had to completely overhaul my life bit by bit and all the way down to the core. I needed a program, something with structure that I could follow that would help me transform. So, I created a health and well-being program that I would test and tweak for years to come called the **Three to Be™ Program.** I researched why my medical issues kept happening to me and what the lessons were in all of it. Everything I knew (or thought I knew) about my health up to that time, I chucked right out the window. Buh-bye and good riddance! With gusto in my soul, I began changing my perspective on health to one that was holistic, a.k.a. whole-body.

WHY I HAD TO CREATE THE THREE TO BE™ PROGRAM

One of the greatest skills my parents passed along to my siblings and me was the importance of having structure. That allowed us to be incredibly focused and get things done. Flexibility was important, of course, but structure was necessary to create a sense of stability and balance in life. As education is paramount in our Indian culture, my parents taught us how to structure our learning by creating schedules and routines and grouping items into small tasks to get them done. By doing this, we achieved our learning goals and felt accomplished, but more importantly, we were driven to move on to the next stage. For example, every day after we finished dinner, my mother made my sister and I take turns running through our times tables from one to 20. And she'd time us: "One times one equals one; one times two equals two," and so on. If we missed a number, we'd literally have to go back to one times one! Only when we were done could we pick up our plate and leave the dinner table. I absolutely hated that ritual! But it led to me enrolling in advanced placement classes in freshman year. (That may have been mom's plan all along, although it seemed Asian Tiger Mom-ish at the time.)

The only way I knew I could go about achieving my North Star was to create a step-by-step program that I could follow in order to achieve my goal. For their part, my parents believed I needed a mantra, or a set of words in Sanskrit that practitioners believe have psychological and/or spiritual powers. The word "mantra" actually comes from two Sanskrit words: "MAN" means mind and "TRA" means vehicle or instrument. So, a mantra is an instrument of the mind, a powerful sound or vibration you can use to transport the mind from a state of activity to one of stillness and deep meditation. Using mantras can help break through subconscious barriers to evoke true positive change. I thought of my mantra as a tagline made up of three components that would act as the main categories that would resonate throughout my life.

In my youth, I remember a conversation amongst my mom and aunties around what their wishes were for their kids. My mom stated that first and foremost, she was grateful for having healthy children. And she always wanted us to be safe, out of harm's way, and to prosper in life. That conversation popped up in my head weeks after I had left the emergency room. I loved everything about those three notions and felt connected to them.

And so those themes of health, safety, and prosperity became the mantras and tenets I would live by going forward. In creating the *Three to Be*™ *Program*, I developed a set of actionable, repeatable steps that bring value at each stage and are embedded in the principles of **Be Healthy, Be Safe + Be Well**™. Creating and following these steps has allowed me to completely transform my life, love myself, and thrive. But as we'll explore later in this book, I also wanted others to be able to learn from my experiences, so the *Three to Be*™ *Program* needed to be easy and affordable enough to be doable by others. As everyone's North Star is personalized, the *Three to Be*™ *Program* is designed to work as a mix-and-match plan that allows you to achieve your definition of optimal health.

THE NET NET

Even with a plan on a page, I still went to bed every night saying a little prayer that one day my food allergies would be gone. I didn't care how it happened—I just wished they would disappear magically overnight, as sudden as winning the lottery. Luck would have a part in that wish, because in 2020—after a decade of working my *Three to Be*™ *Program* rigorously—test results showed that all of my food allergies had been eliminated. *All* of them. They were gone. No more. Sayonara! The cherry on top was that my asthma had also gone dormant. At times, I still cannot articulate how shocked yet joyous I felt when I heard that news.

BECAUSE FOR THE FIRST TIME SINCE THE AGE OF THREE, I WAS AND STILL AM ALLERGY-FREE!

All of the research, testing, and changes I undertook to transform my health and well-being after my 2008 incident led me to write this book. I wrote this as a gift to myself to chronicle all I have been through and how I have evolved into a beautiful human that I love. But I also wrote this for people who are still dealing with daily issues related to food and want to transform their own health holistically. This includes anyone who wants to get healthy, lose weight, and/or manage their food allergies, and it also includes all those who are dealing with food-related diseases such as diabetes. In each chapter to come, I tell my own story and outline the steps you can take to get started on your journey. At the essence of my transformation and this book is the ability to look inward with a deep lens, strategizing, journaling, testing, and tweaking to gain insights and to take different actions going forward.

For most of my life, I had done an outstanding job of keeping my food allergies and asthma hidden from the rest of the world...at least, until my hand was forced. In reading my personal stories, trials, and tribulations, I hope to inspire and encourage you to look at your own well-being holistically and through a lens of discovery, prevention, love, and kindness. *Three to Be™ Program* is about defining what optimal health means to you and designing your life to achieve it. Almost dying allowed me to awaken to life. If I can do it, so can you!

The year 2008 was my rock bottom, and the only place I could go from there was up. This is how I did it.

PART 1

Awakening

ONE

The Last Supper

I n late 2008, I arrived home to San Francisco from a two-week business trip to China and Hong Kong. I met up with 12 close friends for happy hour drinks that turned into a late dinner at one of our fave Asian restaurants. It was somewhere we had been to many times before, and it had a great ambiance: dim lighting, lounge music, sexy cocktails and people, and smells of scrumptious food that would make any heart skip a beat. As the guest of honor, I was strategically placed in the middle of a long, rectangular table. I joked to our crew that we resembled Leonardo da Vinci's mural *The Last Supper* depicting Jesus with his Apostles.

Over the years, whenever this close group went out for dinner, I had taken on the duty of ordering all of the food for the table. I had learned and perfected individual preferences, and besides, and no one wanted to deal with relaying my food allergies to the server. That night, I ordered a bunch of appetizers and entrées that we were going to share family-style. As I did so, I emphasized to the server that we absolutely could *not* have any nuts or nut oils like peanut oil in any of the dishes due to my food allergies. He wrote down some notes and threw me an understanding look while saying, "Okay, okay, no nuts."

I then declared half-jokingly, "Listen, people, don't be mixing spoons and forks in the dishes! I'd like to live another day." This was my way of telling my friends not to cross-contaminate anything, as my Spidey sense overheard one friend order a side salad and tell the server it was just for him, so it was okay to keep the nuts on it. Appetizers and

cocktails started flowing as the sound of clinking glasses rang in celebration that I was home.

During dinner, I felt a tingling sensation all over my body that said,
"Life is great!" After coming off of one of the best trips I'd ever had in
my life and eating some of the greatest Asian food in the world, I was
incredibly happy to be home and surrounded by people whom I loved
dearly. In both China and Hong Kong, I had gorged on dumplings, rice
noodles, hotpots, and other delicacies with the help of Mr. Lee, the
general manager of our China office, who had traveled with us and
had become my official translator for all things food allergy.

As we continued to the main courses, the tingling feeling became
more prominent. I lifted up my blouse sleeves and looked at my arms,
but I didn't see anything wrong, so I continued to eat. As time passed
and the tingling became a feeling of internal itchiness, I busted out my
compact mirror to look at my face. Then I asked my friend sitting next
to me, "Hey, do you see anything on my face?"

"Just a gorgeous smile, babe! You okay?" she replied.

"Oh, I'm just feeling a bit itchy. But no red anything on my face,
right?" I asked.

She said no and added that perhaps the jet lag was hitting me and
I just needed a good night's sleep. She was absolutely right.

"I think I'll pop a Benadryl® to stop feeling itchy, but then my clock
will be ticking to get home," I said. What an annoying buzzkill after
such a fun evening!

"Popping a Benadryl®" was something I'd done in the past. Benadryl®
is an antihistamine that's used to relieve allergic symptoms, including
rashes, overall itching, and itchy eyes, nose, and throat. I also knew that
drowsiness was one of the side effects that would set in soon. On top
of that, I had been drinking alcohol, which was a no-no combination
with Benadryl®. Once we finished dinner, I would have to go straight

home and sleep instead of continuing on to after-hours drinks like some of my friends were already discussing doing.

By the time I got home and was ready for bed, the itching was completely unbearable—it was as if a million mosquitoes had decided to bite me all at once, over and over. In my already-altered state, I popped a second Benadryl® approximately one hour after the first in the hopes that I'd sleep soundly and wake up in the morning feeling better. As I got into bed, my body felt super uncomfortable—on top of the itching, my belly was full and bloated from all the salty foods and drinks. I propped up a few pillows to sleep on, placed my dog Snoop right next to me, and immediately conked out.

Around two o'clock in the morning, something suddenly woke me up, like I was having a nightmare. But it wasn't a noise and it wasn't Snoop, who was wrapped around my left arm and fast asleep. It was the worst chest pain I'd ever felt in my life. It felt like someone had lined up a pile of bricks, dropped them onto my chest, and was sitting on top of them, flattening me. My chest hurt like hell. I was wheezing and having trouble freely catching air, so I peeled Snoop off my arm and sat up in bed. Something was wrong. Desperately wrong.

I rolled off my bed and onto the floor. It took every ounce of strength I had to crawl to my bathroom ten feet away. I felt like Leonardo DiCaprio in the scene from *The Wolf of Wall Street* where he was so hopped up on Quaaludes that he had to crawl from his kitchen, out of his house, into his car, and drive himself to the hospital.

When I finally made it to the bathroom and turned on the light, I screamed in horror at what I saw. That sound woke up Snoop, who started barking loudly. I was *covered* in huge red welts that were each approximately one inch in diameter. As I reached up and felt welts all over my scalp, my eyes felt like they were going to pop out of my head in shock; my mouth nearly dropped to the floor. The welts ran down my face, shoulders, arms, back, stomach, legs...all the way to my toes. Not an inch was left uncovered. I stood there naked, unrecognizable, resembling Chet from *Weird Science.* I immediately started crying hysterically, which caused me to hyperventilate.

What I didn't realize until much later was that I was in a delayed state of anaphylaxis. I had probably been in this state before going to bed. Obviously, popping two Benadryl® wasn't going to fix my anaphylaxis, because that's not even what it's for! Having had a bunch of alcoholic drinks wasn't helping my brain function or focus, either.

The first thing I should have done when I saw my hives was to grab my EpiPen® and inject myself. EpiPen® is an auto-injectable device that delivers epinephrine, a life-saving medication used when someone is experiencing a severe allergic reaction, like what was happening to me in that exact moment! But in my hysteria, that notion never even crossed my mind as my EpiPen® was in my still-unpacked luggage. It all hit me so fast that I didn't realize what was actually happening and therefore forgot what to do!

The one thing I did do was find my cell phone. I speed-dialed my older sister, a doctor of pharmacy because she would know what to do! (And by the way, she lives across the country on the East Coast. What was I thinking? Well, I wasn't!) Thank God, she answered and quickly managed to figure out that something very serious was going on. She told me to hold the line while she called 911 from her home phone. Her second frantic call was to my next-door neighbor whom I was great friends with. She told her to go over to my house and get me to the emergency room *now* or I might not make it.

Jenny, a.k.a. my sista-from-another-mista, was sound asleep at the time, but jolted out of bed and reached my apartment within minutes. She started banging on the door as I lay on the floor in my bedroom, fading fast. My sister yelled into the phone for me to get up and let Jenny in;

I cried even more that my sister was yelling at me. But I managed to put on a T-shirt and get to the front door.

My dog—just as hysterical as I was—was barking like mad at the mad person banging on our door at two o'clock in the morning. I slowly opened the door. Wearing only her short T-shirt nightie, Jenny took one look at me and gasped. "Oh, Lawd, have mercy! Oh no gurl! We gots to go," she said in her southern drawl.

She grabbed my arm as I mumbled, "Snoop?"

"I'll come back for him later, but gurl, we got to go *now!*" she said.

She came inside, grabbed a pair of sweatpants and my purse, and gave Snoop a bone to calm him down before helping me into her car. The ambulance never even made it to my house because we were jetting through every red light like *Thelma and Louise* to the nearest emergency room.

The next 36 hours were critical and my longest stay in the emergency room since I had first been diagnosed with food allergies. Jenny stayed by my side, called my parents and other besties, and even took a quick trip back to my house to walk and feed Snoop. Meanwhile, I was hooked up to IVs along with a breathing apparatus to help with my wheezing and asthma. A myriad of medical staff asked me questions and measured the hives on my body. I had so many drugs in my system along with the alcohol that I couldn't move or process anything that was going on.

"Soni, you awake?" Jenny asked me after a few hours. "Gurl, I have never seen nothing like that! You gave me such a scare. You should have seen it! Oh, and I called your parents, and they're freaking out. Your mom said she's gonna kill you."

My parents! OMG! If this episode didn't kill me, *they* certainly were going to when they arrived from the East Coast. They had never been happy about me moving to California and had always been worried that something like this would happen! When I first got the job offer to move to San Francisco, I had told my parents that California was going to heal my food allergies because it was a healing place—at least, according to shows like *Dynasty* that I watched on television as a child. But now this! I was completely and utterly a hot mess.

HITTING ROCK BOTTOM

How the hell had I ended up in the emergency room again? I hadn't had any emergency-room related incidents in the 13 years prior, so I felt like this had come out of nowhere. I was totally crushed to be in the ER again. And this wasn't like any anaphylactic situation I'd had before—this one felt like a Mack truck had hit me and then backed up to run me over a second time. Yet somehow, I had survived both times, although I didn't know why. The words "I should be dead" kept ringing through my head.

Many hours later, the ER attending doctor came into my room and said that Jenny had relayed information that I had bad food allergies. "It looks like you've had a very severe food allergy reaction that started an onset of anaphylaxis. You went into anaphylactic shock. You are incredibly lucky to be alive, thanks to your friend," the doctor told me.

I looked down at my arms and saw that the hives were still there. "Yes, your hives are rather large and haven't dissipated yet," the doctor went on. "I want to make sure they go down a bit with the medication we're giving you before we can speak about releasing you."

When I heard the doctor's diagnosis, I almost laughed. There was no way this could be my food allergies—I had told the server about my nut allergy and there weren't supposed to be nuts whatsoever in any of the dishes. The staff had assured me that they would handle it and the food would be nut-free! The doctor must be mistaken.

"When was the last time you had a severe reaction due to your food allergies?" she asked.

"Thirteen years ago," I said.

"That's quite a bit of time. Do you have an allergy doctor? If so, I want you to meet with him or her in the next few weeks to make sure you don't have any new food or other allergies," she said.

New allergies? Other allergies? The doc must be smoking crack! The thought of *new* food allergies made me want to die. Thirteen years had gone by with no anaphylaxis and no emergent situations that had sent me to the hospital. Of course, I had had some itchy, I-don't-feel-so-well, upset-stomach types of occurrences during that time, but nothing serious and nothing that some Benadryl® couldn't fix. And given that none of those occurrences had been severe during the past 13 years, I had possibly gotten a little lax with my food allergies. So hearing the doctor's diagnosis and that I might have *new* food allergies left me feeling completely defeated.

The doctor also spoke briefly about biphasic anaphylaxis, which is the recurrence of symptoms within one to 72 hours, typically occurring within ten hours after the initial reaction. Biphasic reactions can occur with no other exposure to an allergen, are treated in the same manner as anaphylaxis, and can be more severe than the initial reaction. Given I lived alone with Snoop, she was going to keep me in the hospital for a while. I agreed that was a good idea.

I stayed in the hospital for almost three days, which gave me plenty of time to analyze everything. Was God testing me or trying to teach me some lesson I hadn't gotten right yet? Why had I been allowed to live in good health for a little over a decade? How could I eat in China and Hong Kong without getting sick? After all, their cuisine uses different forms of nuts in most foods. My head was pounding thinking about all of this, but I couldn't turn off my thoughts.

When I was finally ready to be released, I was sent home with a huge bag full of medications, inhalers, and creams to help suppress my hives and asthma. In addition, I received prescriptions, refill scripts, and a reminder note to see my allergist as soon as I felt up to it.

Jenny's eyes popped out of her head like *Beetlejuice* when she peeked inside the bag. "That's a lot of stuff, Soni!" she said, horrified. Sista, ain't that the truth! The regimen I had been given contained 30-plus pills a day taken over four doses. I felt the need to hire an assistant just to tell me which pills to take and when.

Two weeks after I was released from the hospital, the hives were still on my body. Ugh! So I went to see my allergist for a thorough examination. Before I had moved to San Francisco, the two most important things I locked in were 1) the location of the closest emergency room to my apartment and 2) an allergist. After interviewing what felt like a million allergists, like a godsend, I was recommended to the team at The Allergy & Asthma Clinic, and their medical Director, Dr. Andrew C. Engler, M.D. The philosophy at The Allergy & Asthma Clinic was not to continue to restrict the food in my life given I had so many food allergies, but rather to understand the underlying issues that were going on and create a plan that worked for me.

As my allergist poured over my records from the ER, he proceeded to tell me that it seemed like there may have been some cross-contamination in the food at dinner and agreed that I possibly had some new food allergies.

"I don't agree! I think I picked up something in China or Hong Kong, like some bug or something," I said vehemently.

My allergist smiled. (I would go on to learn that he always loved my vigorous attitude.) He said he understood that this information was very hard to process. He repeated that I was very lucky to be alive. "We can answer all of your questions," he reassured me. "Let's start with the one I'm sure is on the top of your mind, which is what's going on with the hives and when will they go away?"

Yes! That was the *only* question on my mind. I don't think I had necessarily expected the hives to be gone immediately, but I had expected them to be gone before I left the hospital. Now here I was almost two weeks *after* the incident, and the hives were still all over my body, pissing me off even more as each hour went by.

My allergist reminded me that the most common type of allergic reaction to food is an IgE-mediated food allergy and that hives are a symptom of this. He also stated that my hives were acute and possibly could be chronic and last a bit longer. The medications I was given in the hospital were to reduce and suppress my symptoms, but it could take time for my hives to fully dissipate given how severe my reaction was. He explained that there was a lot of toxicity in my body and it needed time to heal.

"Like how much time?" I asked.

"It's hard to say. I've seen other patients where it's taken a few weeks or months, or even..." he trailed off.

"Or even what?" I asked impatiently as my blood pressure started to rise.

"Or in the worst cases, up to a year or more," he said.

My entire body froze as the words "Kill me now!" flashed through my head.

My life was crumbling. One minute, I was loving life and happy to be home; the next, I was almost dead. I became convinced that having a severe anaphylaxis incident after 13 years of somewhat good health was God's way of reminding me that he or she could take me out at any time, so I could never be lax when it came to my food allergies. Fine! I wouldn't be lax again. But learning that I potentially had *more* allergies and could have hives for a long time?? Well, that was God telling me I was doing everything wrong. Or at least, I felt that way. And in order to make sure I learned the lesson, I had to go through this trauma a little while longer—like one year! And the funny part is that I'm not even religious.

FOR THE NEXT YEAR OF MY LIFE, I WOKE UP EVERY SINGLE DAY WITH HUGE RED HIVES ALL OVER MY BODY. YES, FOR ONE YEAR.

Three hundred and sixty-five days.

Eight thousand, seven hundred, and sixty hours.

Five hundred and twenty-five thousand, six hundred minutes.

Thirty-one point fifty-four million seconds.

One full year.

When I woke up at 6:30 a.m., they were there. When I went to bed at 11:00 p.m., they were there. When I woke up in the middle of the night to get a glass of water, they were there.

It was official: **I'd hit rock bottom.**

My body was full of medications to suppress hives that were not being suppressed, and my mind, spirit, and emotions felt like they were decaying. Rock bottom wasn't supposed to happen to someone like me! It was more for drug addicts or people who did bad things. But those hives living on my body for such a length of time was a reminder that I was doing life wrong and had to figure out how to change it all.

"The wound is the place where Light enters you"[14] were the beautiful words of the 13th-century Persian poet Rumi. His words would touch my soul as I was about to search for strength and embark upon a journey to figure out how to rise from rock bottom.

RISING UP WITH PURPOSE

Three months after that meeting with my allergist, I was put on heavier medications to suppress the hives because they were still all over my body. My misery had taken on a new form. Western meds are formulated to suppress symptoms rather than get to the root cause and eradicate them, but for some reason, the meds weren't doing that, either. My doctors adjusted the medications and dosages for weeks to find the right combination that could work, and as a side effect, I was left feeling loopy, weak, and depressed. That was not a great place to be seeing as I was already back at work with a full load on my plate.

I felt like I couldn't catch a break and there was no end in sight, so I decided to throw myself a pity party and wallowed in it for months. I knew I needed to find strength in this situation, but I was not ready yet. Everything sucked: the limited foods I could eat, the fact that I was too weak to work out, my work life, and my personal life. I cut out all forms of interactions with other breathing souls except for my dog, which worried my friends. But no one needed to see me looking like a monster—it was bad enough that was what *I* saw when I looked in the mirror. (At some point, I stopped doing that, too.) My plans to possibly create a new venture in food and wine were kiboshed as I thought, "If food hates me, why the hell would I want to start a business with it?" I just needed to be alone for a while and be sad and take inventory of everything that had happened, knowing full well I wasn't going to stay down in the dumps forever.

If I were going to be a hermit crab, the best place to be was surfing the web and stalking what others were doing on social media, because then I could hide behind my laptop without anyone seeing the beast I had become. Post after post on Facebook and Instagram showed the great and exciting times everyone was having as they lived their hive-free lives. That put me even more in the dumps. This was bad. I needed something to slap the depression out of me.

Then one day, I saw these words on a social media post: "You have two choices in life: evolve or repeat." After staring at the post and reading the comments, I wrote down my own quote on a piece of paper: "You have two choices in life: hives or no hives."

I laughed aloud as I stared at my own words. There it was! Something about those words evoked a visceral feeling in my body. In a way, that made me so mad at myself, because I had spent months reading inspirational posts, yet nothing had really resonated with me until now. I had read comment after comment by people who had written about something they had overcome, normal people like you and me. I had gone down a spiral looking into these people's profiles and what they were posting about. So many stories, all unique in their own way... If others out there could overcome their grim situations, then why couldn't I?

Finding that "evolve or repeat" quote was a direct message from the Gods. It was telling me I could choose to be a victim of my situation or forge a new path that was different, better, and free from misery and pain. I looked up the word "survivor" on www.dictionary.com. It defined it as "a person who continues to function or prosper in spite of opposition, hardship, or setbacks".[15] At that time, I was somewhat functioning, but I definitely was not prospering.

So, in the evenings after work and on weekends, I devoured as much media as I could, watching videos, listening to podcasts, and reading books and posts about women who had transformed their lives. I read of famous people like Maya Angelou, who in her adolescence transformed from having been a victim of racism into becoming a self-possessed young woman capable of responding to prejudice. Then I read about Sally Ride, who became the first woman in space in 1983. I read about Ruth Bader Ginsberg, the second woman appointed to the US Supreme Court, who used her voice for dissent and shaped the course of our nation's history. I read about Billie Jean King, a former number one world professional tennis star, and I read about Bethany Hamilton, whose left arm was bitten off by a shark in a surfing accident in 2003 when she was only 13 years old. She went on to place first at the National Scholastic Surfing Association annual competition in 2005. J.K. Rowling battled depression, suicidal tendencies, and poverty to become one of the most beloved British authors in the world for her hugely popular *Harry Potter* series. And of course, I read about Oprah's iconic story.

In February 2008, the US edition of *The Guardian* did an interview with one of my all-time idols, Mary J. Blige, called "I Saw My Life Going Down A Drain".[16] The article stated, "Blige's career can be divided in two: a troubled first half, during which she made her name by working through her problems on record; and a second half in which she has found God, and love, and beaten her addictions. Her new album, *Growing Pains*, seemed at first to fit the pattern of this second period. 'The album's concept is the acceptance that perfection is impossible,' she says. 'It's about balance.'"

Mary J. talked about how "...*Growing Pains* hits hardest when she (Blige) focuses on the imperfection, scratches at the scars of her emotional wounds." In this article, Mary was describing exactly what I was feeling and going through. One of the most powerful statements Blige made in that interview was her reference to another troubled singer, Amy Winehouse. Winehouse's music oozes "I am what I am." Blige stated, "You gotta love a person who says in front of the world: 'This is me; this is who I am.'"

Before 2008, I had never done that. I needed to confront my fears, and not just the fear of eating something that would send me to the emergency room. There were other deep fears instilled in me from childhood, from the experiences I've had to the way people treated me, talked to me, and acted or reacted around me because of my illness. Now it was time to face them all.

The more I educated myself about other people's struggles, the more I began to consider that there was a path for me as a survivor—someone who wouldn't let her food allergies run or ruin her life. But in order to become that survivor, I needed to do everything completely differently. I needed to evolve into something different, stronger, smarter, wiser, and healthier! I had to envision and manifest who I wanted to be. Just like when my computer gave me the spinning mouse wheel, my life needed a reboot.

In the decade following my 2008 incident, I reflected on my life and documented my "why:" who I was, who I wanted to be, and how I was going to achieve it. I thought about negative patterns and how to break them, and I thought about changing the way I lived life and how I could lead a life with purpose. If God was trying to teach me a lesson, I had to figure out what that lesson was so that I would not repeat the mistake. I *never* ever wanted to be on that emergency room table again.

Through years of journaling, reading, researching, participating in focus groups, having discussions with friends, holding sessions with therapists, creating plans, executing plans, and testing and tweaking plans, I realized that this work was the creative outlet I had been looking for. I wanted to share my story of transformation of having had severe food allergies and asthma and then shedding them, to help others out there who are like me thrive.

In his 1982 book *Rejection*, author James R. Sherman wrote about how to overcome rejection. Sherman advised readers not to fixate on the past, making this observation: "You can't go back and make a new start, but you can start right now and make a brand-new ending".[17]

Many realizations came out of my full year in hives. The starting place was realizing that I needed a mission/purpose in life. I needed my North Star so that I could begin looking at the bigger picture. My life was no longer just about my physical health—it had to encompass all parts of the body, mind, spirit, and emotions, because they were all tied together. When one part was down, all of the others were misaligned. I had to be dedicated to this transformation like I'd never been before; it had to become a way of life for me.

Everything I knew from the past about managing my food allergies was over, and I began to learn again with an open mind. When I felt myself falter, I looked at one of the many disgusting photos I had taken of the hives all over my body to remind myself where I could end up if I didn't make changes.

There really aren't words to articulate how I felt waking up every single day for an entire year with big red hives all over my body. It completely broke me. But there was a silver lining in that event! I just had to finally open my eyes and see it.

TWO

East Meets West

To figure out where to begin, I didn't just go back to the events of that night—I went back in the day to when I was first diagnosed with severe food allergies to determine how I had gotten to this point in my life.

My parents emigrated to the United States from India in 1960 to pursue higher education and opportunity. They were adventurers who left their families 8,000 miles away to make it on their own in their new home. But their greatest challenge wasn't trying to fit into a culture of drainpipe jeans, miniskirts, and knee-high go-go boots. Rather, it was how to raise three first-generation American kids and also instill Eastern culture into their lives.

Food was a huge part of that culture. I grew up in a family like the one in the blockbuster 2002 movie *My Big Fat Greek Wedding*. In that movie, the main character, Toula, was constantly surrounded by family, whether she was at work, having a meal, or making a life decision. Their family was a little social network before there was Facebook, gathering at all hours of the night to help one another maneuver through life. While cooking and sharing amazing foods, they dispensed advice that they believed would instantly make all problems go away.

"Having boyfriend troubles, Toula? Let me comfort you with some baba ghanoush, pita bread, and 12 kabobs!" her mother would say. Food was the main component of solving all issues for Toula's family, and it was in mine as well. Just like Toula's, my family is big, and always up in your business. Many of us are amazing cooks who take the time and effort to create scrumptious flavors to share. To my family, food is defined by a few fundamentals: it has to be delicious, beautiful, creative, and made with intention. That means not only does the dish need to make sense from a flavor perspective, the cook's heart and soul must be *felt* in the dish. In the 1980s, the media coined us as being "foodies," and we rejoiced!

Foodies are people who don't just like to eat—foodies seek out new food experiences wherever they go. They are particular and opinionated about ingredients and flavors in dishes and like to discuss them in depth, probably over the meal you're eating with them. Foodies come in all shapes and sizes and are passionate people who like to chow down and share with others. They have a general attitude of "At our table, the more, the merrier!" This was the essence of my upbringing.

Not only do I like to eat, but I've been in the kitchen helping my mom since I could walk. Our kitchen was an exciting place full of wonderful smells where things happened fast. And I got to taste everything! Culturally, Indian girls always help their mothers in the kitchen, from cooking to setting the table to helping wash dishes and clean up. I always enjoyed being in the kitchen with my mom as I sat at the table and rolled chapati, or homemade flat wheat bread. Then I would watch as she put it on a tava (a cast-iron griddle) to cook it, where it would puff up and then flatten out. My eyes would widen with excitement as she put the chapati on a plate, slathered homemade ghee and some sugar onto it, and then rolled it up like a taquito. It was my special treat just for helping her in the kitchen as a young child. And it was everything to me.

AN EXOTIC WORLD OF DINNER PARTIES

The million-dollar question every day at breakfast was "So what should we have for dinner?" And with this question, our day began. My parents had grown up eating all of their meals together as a family sitting at the dinner table. There were no iPads, cell phones, or gamers at the time—you just had old-fashioned conversations with your parents and invited friends. You talked about your day at school and what you learned, and you definitely ate everything on your plate. No questions.

When my parents moved to the US, they settled down in Philadelphia, Pennsylvania and met many young Indian couples just like them, couples who had left their families to live in America as well. Over time, these friends became family to my parents. They were like an OG crew—they did everything together, from traveling to going to restaurants to hosting dinner parties. At these dinner parties, homemade Indian food was served and provided everyone with the feeling of being close to their far-away families.

Their crew all started having kids around the same time, and they continued their dinner party extravaganzas with all us kids in tow. There were about 20 of us who were approximately one year apart; many were the same age. Imagine growing up with that many built-in siblings! I quickly forgot about my middle child syndrome, because I no longer was one. My "fake cousins," as we called each other, surrounded me and made me feel special. I feel so incredibly blessed to have grown up this way and experienced so many things in life with my huge extended family.

My parents hosted dinner parties four to five times per week. I have no idea how they did it after coming home from a long day at work. But being surrounded by people they loved and sharing meals was embedded into who they are, so they never saw it as a chore. And the food that would come out of their kitchen was better than any James Beard-winning restaurant you'd ever eat at.

My parent's dinner parties were epic, all-hands-on-deck events. Dad always assumed the front of the house role, making sure the ambiance was perfect from the get-go, including the music, cocktails, and lighting. He would even pop into the kitchen to be the unofficial taste-tester of what was to come. Meanwhile my mom, a.k.a. Wonder Woman, took care of everything else: cooking, cleaning as she cooked, and watching over us kids while lecturing us about something or other.

Like a rooster, my father would sit perched at the entrance to our home, making sure guests were greeted with a single malt scotch (which he would already be partaking in). Mom would be in the kitchen frying up five-spice shrimp for appetizers, stirring a pot of kolhapuri mutton curry for dinner, and checking on her ras malai, a traditional dessert made with paneer...all at the same time! Mom looked like the Hindu goddess Lakshmi, the goddess of wealth, prosperity, and luck who had multiple arms and could do anything.

As guests would arrive and the adults socialized in the house, we kids would play in the backyard until we all sat down at the dinner table together. Similar to what her parents had decreed, mom had one simple rule for me and my sister: "Whatever is put on your plate must disappear." This was not an idle threat, and I so longed for a family dog to feed my vegetables to when I was growing up! She made us sit at the table for hours until that last bite was gone. Having grown up in India and seen so much poverty across the country, my parents were very conscious of food waste. They often reminded us that most kids in India didn't even get one meal a day and that we were extremely blessed to get several.

Once the dinner parties started, it was like fairy dust and magic: people talking over each other at 110 decibels, passing plates, pouring drinks, speaking different languages. And boy, was there a lot of laughter! Over the years, I learned valuable information at the dinner table, sometimes more than I did at school. For example, I learned dirty worlds and how to tell dirty jokes in Marathi, our native language, and also in Hindi. I also learned that most adults at the table didn't understand the rules of NFL football, yet heatedly debated how well the Philadelphia Eagles would do that season. The food we ate was also always a topic of conversation as aunties would try to learn my mom's innermost secrets of what she put into each dish and how it turned out so good.

"Oh, saffron? Huh. Interesting... I mean, it tastes very good, but who would think to put saffron in this dish?" an auntie would ask.

Mom and I always looked at each other and smiled at backhanded compliments like those. From the men, you'd only hear moans and grunts of pleasure, because they were incredibly happy to eat a meal that reminded them of their mother's cooking. If my father loved a particular dish, he would say "Fabulous!" He'd repeat the word after almost every bite. "Fabulous! Um-hmm, fabulous... I mean, this is fabulous!"

Most of the time, the food we ate was Indian food. But my mom learned to master many other cuisines to pacify her American kids, who annoyed her by begging to eat Hostess brands Ding Dongs for dinner. As time went by, she expanded her own cooking skills into homemade Italian, Chinese, and even Filipino food to add variety and expand our palates.

Those dinner parties were beautiful chaos in their own way, and I feel very lucky to have been exposed to so many people and so much culture since birth. They gave me an appreciation for food and for the community that has stuck with me all of my life. Our kitchen was the heart of our home, and over the years, many people came in and out of our home to share food, stories, and love. I grew up rooted in family, culture, and food, all of which gave me a beautiful foundation for life. And I am so grateful for it.

PB&J: THE SANDWICH OF DEATH

One particular dinner party in the 1970s set off a chain of events that would stay with us forever—a sort of urban legend in our community.

As the kids were playing in the backyard before dinner, a plate of tea-sized samosas (a fried Indian snack with a savory filling of spiced potatoes, onions, and peas) and some other sandwiches were placed on the table for us to share. I was around three-and-a-half years old and happily playing near the swing set as I was handed a sandwich to snack on. A few bites was all my body needed for the chaos to begin.

Big red welts immediately appeared on my body, and I started choking. Between the loud music coming from the house and the kids screaming at what they were seeing, it could have been game over for me. It took some quick thinking from the adults—most of whom were actually doctors—to decipher the commotion, put me into a car, and rush me to our local emergency room. That night's dinner party came to a screeching halt.

In the emergency room, my parents watched in horror as their little girl was hooked up to IV fluids and breathing apparatuses and pumped with medications to save her life. I almost died that day on the emergency room table. As my twenty-something-year-old immigrant parents watched helplessly through the glass window in the emergency room, their lives changed forever.

During my hospital stay, I was diagnosed with severe food allergies, and I was also placed on several medications to suppress the symptoms of anaphylactic shock caused by the peanut butter and jelly sandwich I had eaten in the backyard.

In the months following that incident, my doctors conducted many tests to determine which exact foods I was allergic to and if there was anything else wrong with me. Alas, there was! We found out I also had environmental allergies, asthma, and allergies to penicillin, Keflex, and erythromycin. The bad news continued to pile up, as did the stress on us as a family. I was definitely the star of the siblings and getting all kinds of attention from my parents even when I didn't want it. This was much to the dismay of my older sister, who had always been the shining star of the family.

My doctors gave us some key pieces of information soon after my food allergy diagnosis:

- I might acquire more food allergies as I age.

- My food allergies could get worse over time.

- Genetically, I could be predisposed to other ailments.

But it was these additional statements that felt like the final nails in my coffin:

- The exact cause of food allergies is still unknown.

- There is no cure for food allergies.

- Food allergies could result in death.

All of the above would come true later in my life. Indeed, as I've gotten older, my body has acquired more food allergies like a bad habit.

AT THE PEAK IN 2008, I WAS DIAGNOSED WITH OVER 32 FOOD ALLERGIES, ADDING RANDOM ITEMS SUCH AS CORN, HALIBUT, AND AVOCADO TO MY LIST.

My allergies absolutely did get worse over time, meaning each emergent situation I had was worse than the previous one had been. Some of my allergies, like avocado, were also topical—if I touched an avocado, my hands broke out in hives. And as I got older, whenever I had an allergic reaction, the length of time it took me to recover seemed to get longer and longer. It was incredibly scary to think about how I would be able to manage all of this as I aged.

CREATING A "ME" PLAN

For most of my life, I was told that in order to manage my food allergies, I had to control what I was eating and take Western meds. Not really a great overall plan, but it sufficed for many years. With the help of my team of doctors, soon after my diagnosis, we came up with a "ME plan." That stood for "medication" and "eating." Taking medications was the only treatment option I was given, and my eating plan had one specific goal: "Do not eat anything you are allergic to." I was told to strictly avoid all forms of peanuts and tree nuts or risk going into anaphylaxis again. We had to ask for a full list of tree nuts since there are many varieties in the United States. In order for me to stay safe, I also had to *not* eat things that obviously had nuts in them, such as peanut butter, pecan pie, or nut candies.

Reading food labels became a new part of our daily life. Yes, in the 1970s, my parents were reading food labels! We learned that an ingredient could have several names, plus there were also nut oils and nut flours to consider. On top of that, my body might react differently to the raw versus cooked form of a food. It really was just too much all at once, because we also had to deal with learning about my environmental allergies to things like dust and mold *and* we had to deal with my asthma. My family suffered through all of this together, with my parents repeatedly calling *their* parents back in India to keep them up to date. None of our family in India had ever heard of food allergies—they believed it was something the US had given me. It took me years and several more ER visits before I concluded that they were right!

The eating part of the ME plan was made up of homemade Indian food and a mix of Western foods for the relentless American kid in me. My mom wasn't a boxed-mashed-potatoes kind of girl, especially when she started reading labels and seeing ingredients such as maltodextrin and sodium caseinate, so she began making everything from scratch. That was an incredibly huge effort. She sometimes added her Indian flair to American dishes, spicing up the homemade mashed potatoes, soups and noodle dishes to break up my monotony.

From the 1970s through the 1990s, conversations around food allergies or the effects of foods on our bodies were scarce compared to what they are today. Back then, we weren't questioning what was in our food or why it was there. There was little awareness, structure, or regulation around food labeling or the quality of ingredients at that time. Food was an industry driven by marketing, with brands stating "wholesome," "nutritious," and "good for you" in large, bold letters on the packaging. Who were we as consumers to question this? My family wasn't looking at food as big business; they did the best they could given the information they had at the time.

As I continued to get older, my mom enforced strict limitations on many American foods I loved to eat (like candy, chips, and soda) because of ingredients with long names that she knew nothing about. But she didn't want to force my diet upon everyone else in the house, so she kept some of my no-no items high on top of the refrigerator. I was gutted watching my siblings gobble down a SNICKERS® whenever they wanted. My copious amounts of crying did not win me a green light to eat even nut-free candies—my mom was not taking any chances. "Better to be safe than sorry" was her motto.

When I started going to school, Mom sent me with homemade Indian food in my Strawberry Shortcake™ lunchbox because she was convinced that the foods she knew and had grown up with were the safest bets. As everyone pulled out their ham and cheese sandwiches with Cheetos or Bugles on the side, I pulled out chicken curry and rice. I felt like Hester Prynne in *The Scarlet Letter*, except in my story, "A" was for "allergies."

The downside of the ME plan was that everyone started to treat me like a delicate china doll, as if even sneezing near me would make me break out in hives. (The plan I was on at the time was about suppressing my symptoms rather than ridding me of my food allergies.) So much of my childhood became trial and error, because none of us had a Ph.D. in food science to know what every single ingredient was. As a result, without trying, I stood out like a sore thumb after my diagnosis. There was nothing I could do about it. Well, until I entered my teenage years and rebelled like hell against everything, including my food allergies.

REBEL WITHOUT A CAUSE

From the ages of three to 12, my parents took the lead and handled everything when it came to my food allergies. But when I turned 13, all bets were off! ...Or at least in my mind, I wanted them to be. Teenage years are about learning, development, and physical changes. The only things I cared about were if I was cool, if I was going to get invited to the cool parties, and who would be the recipient of my first kiss. I wanted to be free from my food allergies and out from under my parents' helicopter. I had already spent one decade living with severe health issues and had had multiple incidents in the emergency room, and I was spent! I just wanted to turn it all off with a magic wand.

Due to the feelings of inadequacy and shame that come along with being a tween in America, I didn't use my voice to speak up about my food allergies...yet I was annoyed with my parents if they did it on my behalf. Television shows and my fave magazines helped this attitude because they made me compare myself to their definition of a beautiful woman, which I was not. I had changes going on with my body, skin, and weight; even my nose seemed to be developing in a way I didn't want. Health issues and body issues were like a one-two punch that affected my mind, spirit, and emotions just as I was trying to somehow fit in. So, I did what any normal teenager would have done in my shoes: I hid my sickness from everyone.

As a family, we did not sit around and discuss our feelings like we saw American families do on television. Instead, we discussed food. I wasn't running to my parents to tell them about some bully or that I felt inadequate compared to other girls in school. Rather, I choose to keep all of that inside or tell a fake cousin, which somehow always had a way of getting back to my parents eventually. When my parents did find out, they fixed the issue rather than sitting down with me and discussing how the situation made me feel. "Who doesn't like you? Tell me now!" was a question I would receive from my parents. Feelings are culturally nonexistent in Indian families. You're just supposed to shove them inside and hope they don't pop out at the wrong time.

One summer during a family trip to India, one of mom's sisters asked me "Soni, why do you have the worries of the world on your face? You're so young! You will get wrinkles."

God, she saw right through me. Living with food allergies and constantly worrying about every damn thing took a toll on me. I was 14 when this happened, and I had been dealing with severe health issues and adolescence all at the same time, which wasn't a pretty picture. Questions would always race through my mind in a blur: "Should I eat it? Will it kill me? What will people think? Do I care?" And of course, the famous question of "Why me?" I never verbalized these—instead, I allowed them to decay me from the inside out.

My parents had done so much for me since my diagnosis that I didn't want to add more stress to their lives by telling them that I too was carrying a burden. At times, I felt like it was literally driving me nuts, no pun intended. I worried about everything in silence. Perhaps I was too young to get wrinkles on my face, but I'm sure this was not healthy behavior.

My teenage years were also a time where I was trying to come to terms with the two sides of my life: Eastern versus Western. I wasn't quite sure that I wanted a balance between them, and for many years I renounced being Indian in favor of being American and trying to fit into the country I was born in. Yet it was that same country that had defined me as "different" because of the color of my skin, my culture, and my food allergies.

My Eastern life was all about family and values and acknowledging that yes, I *was* different and so I didn't need to try to be the same as others (meaning my American friends). But I didn't want to hear the "Love who you are!" messaging from my parents at that time. Those years were very difficult for them as well. They didn't really understand what their kids were going through because they hadn't grown up in the United States. We, on the other hand, couldn't always relate to my parents' way of thinking because we hadn't grown up in India. The mounting pressure of being part of "both sides" was tearing me down. Forcing me to choose a side made me become reckless about my situation.

In high school, the cafeteria sold many items for breakfast, most of which I didn't eat. But can one really turn away from the buttery smells of piping-hot, chocolate-glazed and vanilla-frosted donuts each morning? My mom made sure we ate breakfast at home every day, but my new high school friends and I had a daily ritual of meeting at 7:30 a.m., buying a donut and coffee, and catching up on gossip before heading off to first period. It was our early version of the television show *Gossip Girl*; we even had a pecking order, from the queen bee to the minions. Everyone ate the donuts except me, which at some point became noticeable.

"Do you not like donuts?" my friend asked.

I either said I was watching my weight or that they didn't agree with me. But God, how I drooled, wanting to eat one and fit in with everyone else.

I dared not ask the lunch ladies questions about nuts in donuts or what oil was in the fryer, as I was scared to do this in front of friends who didn't know anything about my food allergies. My options became lying to my friends or coming clean. I chose to lie. Then one day I was put on the spot when the queen bee treated everyone at the table to an assortment of donuts and coffee for her birthday. There were all sorts of varieties, including chocolate and vanilla with nuts on top. Internally, I freaked out.

"There's one with your name on it, Sonia! You have to eat it, or I'll be mad that I wasted money on you. You can be first to pick," she said.

And there it was: teenage peer pressure. I stared at the donuts, thinking it was a bad situation. But as all eyes were on me, I grabbed a chocolate-glazed donut with nuts all over the top, wiped some of the nuts away, and popped the nut-free part into my mouth.

I died and went to heaven. Not literally! But it tasted like a butter paradise: doughy, greasy wondrousness coated my entire mouth. I even got a "Yay!" from the table as everyone went about their eating.

And then as if in slow motion, my older sister walked into the cafeteria with her posse of friends. In a panic, I spat my donut into a napkin and put the rest in my bag to throw away later. This did not go unnoticed by my friends; later, I told them that I didn't love the taste of donuts. Thank God I did not have a reaction that day! I couldn't believe it. I wanted to tell my parents the amazing news, but I couldn't, because they certainly would have killed me. But how was it that I had literally had something with nuts in my mouth and nothing happened? Perhaps I was getting over my food allergies? Or maybe it was just wishful thinking.

That wasn't the only time in high school I took chances. Did I ever get sick? Yes, of course! Reactions manifested immediately or as a delayed reaction. My parents couldn't understand what had happened, because I wouldn't tell them if I had eaten something I shouldn't have. "I don't know" was my go-to answer. Hives appeared many times, and I would pop a Benadryl® as my drug of choice if my chest didn't feel right. Taking chances gave me a euphoric feeling that I was young, wild, and free! I was on top of the world, and nothing could harm me, not even my food allergies. I definitely had some luck on my side during that time.

THE BANANA INCIDENT

In 1995, my senior year of college, I walked into my eight o'clock a.m. Fundamentals of Materials lecture and started choking. Then I slowly went into anaphylactic shock in front of 300 students. Talk about trying to get out of your pop quiz! And it was all because of one measly banana.

I had eaten many bananas in my life without issue, especially before going for a long run. On that day, my college roomie had reminded me to grab a banana on the way to class because we needed to finish them before they went bad. I kindly obliged...and now I was choking in front of the hot guy sitting right in front of me. Mortifying!

A student called 911 as I turned purple. I was rushed to the emergency room at the University of Pennsylvania Hospital. Ironically, that's where I was born; all the way there, I thought, "If it's gonna end now, there is no other place I'd rather die than the place I was born." But I survived and was diagnosed with a banana allergy soon thereafter. My life had officially hit the comical stage.

The Banana Incident of '95 was my only emergent situation during college, and I never told my parents about it. Why? Because I had nightmares that they would force me to move home and commute in my last year so that they could watch over me. (My parents are probably reading this right now and saying, "What?? She almost died eating a banana in 1995 and she didn't tell us? We'll kill her!")

College is one of the most exciting times in someone's life, but it can also be a rocky road, especially for someone with food allergies. On my own for the first time, I realized that I wasn't really managing my food allergies— I was only somewhat speaking up about them and only in certain circumstances. For the most part, I was still in my hiding phase because of shame.

For someone who's never had great luck, my luck started to change in 1998 when I was recruited by a tech startup and moved to sunny California. My dreams of a healthy lifestyle in California were looking like a real possibility! My parents almost had a heart attack when I told them I had accepted a job in San Francisco and would be moving across the country. There were a lot of "Hai, Ram!" phrases thrown around, which in our language means "Oh, God!"

"Hai, Ram, you're doing *whaaat*? Who told you that you could go? Who is hiring you? Do they know about your food allergies? How will you eat? Who will take care of you?" My mother would ask all of these questions in one fell swoop. The only thing that came out of my father's mouth was "NO."

But I was set on leaving behind the life I had lived thus far. In deciding to move to California, I was leaving my food allergies, years of sickness, feelings of shame, and isolation all behind. And I was especially leaving behind the years of someone else telling me what to do and how to do it. I wasn't running away...or was I? I had dreams that living on the East Coast was like living in a cesspool that made me sick and that the West Coast was going to miraculously make me healthy. It seemed like the perfect place, one far enough away to accomplish a life with no food allergies. Nothing was going to stop me from going! *Nothing.*

After I moved to San Francisco, I did all of the things young folks do: I worked hard, traveled, and ate out with friends while avoiding peanuts, tree nuts, and bananas. I didn't forget about my food allergies; I just concentrated on living my new life. It had been three years since my banana incident of 1995, and for the first time, I felt hope. For most of my life, I had been traumatized by the constant worry of eating. Perhaps now San Francisco would remove the dark clouds above me and give me permission to live normally, without food allergies.

And then as if the Universe had answered my prayers, for 13 years after my banana incident of '95, I didn't have a single trip to the emergency room. None. Nada. Zip. I didn't have any nosebleeds, my asthma was under control thanks to the steroid inhalers I was still taking daily, and I rarely even had to pop a Benadryl®. For the first time in my life, something had changed. Someone was finally watching over me and answering my prayers. Was California healing me like I thought it would?

I deemed this time as being the "Lucky 13." As year after year went by and I didn't get sick, I gained confidence. I still was doing allergy testing every year to two years, and my results were constant and horrible, showing that I still had very severe food allergies that needed to be managed. But somehow, they were not manifesting. Nothing was going to stop me from living my life to the fullest for the first time ever! Being sick for so long and then having a random period of time where everything miraculously went in my favor—well, it's like I totally forgot that I had any issues to begin with. I was over the moon!

But as you already know, my Lucky 13 came to a screeching stop in 2008, and my life has never been the same since.

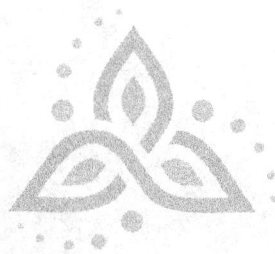

THREE

Designing the Three to Be™ Program

After the events of 2008, I set out to transform my life. I knew full well that achieving my North Star of ridding myself of food allergies would not happen overnight, but I prayed it would happen in my lifetime. My head was in the right game now, and I was giving it my all, no holds barred. It was time for me to take charge, step up to a new level, and figure out some very important aspects of my health and how my health affected my overall life. I referred to this time period as "designing my life."

Author Susan Ariel Rainbow Kennedy (also known as SARK) once said, "Invent your world. Surround yourself with people, color, sounds, and work that nourish you".[18] "Nourishment" was a key word that I seemed to be missing in my life. I needed to carefully and tactically create a plan for what I wanted to achieve, why I wanted to achieve it, and how I would.

I wrote my North Star statement in black, non-erasable ink on a whiteboard in my house. For the first time, I felt like I had vision. I stared at my North Star every day and let it begin to embed into my soul. My next step was to define my "why," i.e., *why* I was working toward my particular North Star. The reason might have seemed obvious: getting rid of my food allergies meant I would be healthy and stay out of the hospital. But that wasn't necessarily the whole "why." I was also looking for a reason why reactions kept happening to me, because four times in an anaphylaxis situation was over the top and quite enough. Defining my "why" needed to be the fire in my soul that would make me come alive and drive me to achieve my North Star. My "why" would not let anything stop me. It had to come from a deep place, and it had to be about more than just my food allergies—it had to be about the way I lived my life, because I could never go back to where I had been.

First, I researched, read books, and scoured social media to look for others like me and understand what struggles they had been through. Through this exercise, I found a few interesting bits of information:

- Many food allergy foundations in the United States conduct research on allergies, provide educational tools, and raise awareness about the disease and how to manage it. Foundations such as the Food Allergy Research & Education organization, the Food Allergy and Anaphylaxis Connection Team, and the Asthma and Allergy Foundation of America fall into this category.

- Physicians have written multitudes of medical websites, books, and articles regarding food and environmental allergies as well as asthma. In these works, physicians discuss the body's reactions and give medical advice on how to take care of yourself to prevent a reaction.

- Several parenting groups swap stories of their children who have severe food allergies and look to share information on how to manage the disease.

- Hundreds of books have been written about food allergies, from cookbooks focused on allergy-friendly recipes to children's stories that deal with managing allergies.

It was amazing to learn about all of these passionate people looking to help one other. I decided that part of my "why" needed to be about helping others like me who suffer on a daily basis and who want to learn how to survive and thrive. When I was first diagnosed, my family did not know a single person who had food allergies. Then, by the time I was nine, my one-year-old first cousin was diagnosed with severe eczema and later would find out that he also had severe food allergies. That was it: just the two of us. As a family, we were still on our own trying to figure everything out with our doctors, because in the '70s and '80s, there was no social media and there were no meetups for parents who had children with food allergies. Contrast that with today: I literally cannot go out for a meal without someone at the table telling the server about their dietary restrictions, whether they are medical restrictions or preferences such as choosing to not eat carbs to keep their weight down.

One of my fave motivational authors, Diego Pérez, once said, "Time does not heal all wounds. It gives them space to sink into our subconscious, where they will still impact your emotions and behavior. What heals is going inward, loving yourself, accepting yourself, listening to your needs, addressing your attachments and emotional history, learning how to let go and follow your intuition".[19] This was so true in my situation! As I was embarking on a journey to heal myself, I inherently knew that I needed to share in detail what I was going through with others in the hopes that it might help them with their own struggles.

So, I wrote down my "why" on the whiteboard:

To empower people with food restrictions to thrive in health and life.

How was I going to empower people? Well, first I had to become empowered about my own health; then I could show others how I had done it. I began to think of myself as a guide or a curator—someone who would do the research and go through the testing and bring back that information to others so that they could make their own decisions.

Throughout the years, I've met thousands of people around the world who have some form of food restrictions. A common thread amongst these people is that they are afraid—afraid of eating, speaking up, traveling, and dating, to name a few things. Fear was driving many facets of their lives, as it had for me for many years. This notion took me back to Mary J. Blige's interview where she had spoken of fear. Fear caused people to not advocate for themselves out of the fear of what others might think. This accurately described my situation for all of the years prior to 2008.

I once dated a guy who had a love/hate relationship with garlic. He loved it, yet every time he'd eat garlic, he would always end up with gas and sometimes diarrhea. When we'd dine out, he would tell the server he was allergic to garlic, which would piss me the hell off. I have zero tolerance for anyone who lies to a restaurant and says they have a food allergy when they don't. It makes it so much worse for people like me who actually do! I asked him if he'd ever seen a doctor about this issue, and his answer was no. So, he was restricting something he loved because of a self-diagnosis, yet he'd never seen a doctor to know for sure if it was an allergy or was caused by something else...!

He was a great example of someone who feared speaking up and explaining the situation to the server because he was embarrassed. If he was trying to impress me, I wasn't impressed, nor was I impressed when his bowels were making all kinds of noises from the bathroom later on.

Fear sucks! It's an ugly hydra of a monster, and something I had dealt with my entire life. It forbade me from really living life, because I was always scared about what I was eating and then I never told anyone about how I felt. But if I were going to chart a path toward my North Star, then no more of that! Everything was about to change. I was going to take all of the bad and the ugly from the previous decades and turn it into a thriving life, and I was going to document it all.

With that thought, I went back to my whiteboard and started sketching out the *Three to Be™ Program*, which was all about "how" I was going to do this.

WHAT IS THE THREE TO BE™ PROGRAM?

The conversation I had with my parents about mantras led me to the three main principles of the *Three to Be™ Program*:

Be Healthy, Be Safe + Be Well™

These principles felt right in my core because I wanted all three of these things in my life! In my mind, I had to elevate them as tenets in order to achieve my North Star. They would be prioritized above and beyond everything else in my life. I did not write these steps as a 1+2=3, per se. Instead, achieving my North Star meant I had to accomplish *all three* of them.

> **THE** *THREE TO BE™ PROGRAM* **WAS GOING TO BE A HOLISTIC PLAN FOR ME TO BE PHYSICALLY, MENTALLY, SPIRITUALLY, AND EMOTIONALLY HEALTHY, SAFE, AND WELL.**

With geeky excitement, I wrote *Be Healthy, Be Safe + Be Well*™ on my whiteboard underneath my North Star. I also wrote it on a yellow sticky note that I stuck on my bathroom mirror so that I could embed those main principles into my brain every day. Then I let them sit in my mind for two weeks without editing them. At the end of that time, everything in my being knew I had found the right path forward.

From 2010 to 2019, I devised, tested, and tweaked steps within each of the three principal areas of the *Three to Be™ Program*. The matrix became a 3x3, where there are three main principles of health, safety, and wellness united with three steps within each principle. The name of the program reflects the desired end result "to be" healthy, safe, and well in order to be free of food allergies, and the trauma associated with them. The steps in this program were designed to allow me to thrive in my health and in my life. I needed to create something that was easy for me and anyone that I would share this program with, like you!

STEPS OF THE THREE TO BE™ PROGRAM

This diagram gives you an easy layout of each of the steps in this 3x3 program. In each of the upcoming chapters, I'll go into detail about each step, why that step was important, how I went about it, and my results. I will also give you recommendations on how you can get started on your own journey to transformation to *Be Healthy, Be Safe + Be Well™* by using the *Three to Be™ Program*.

My wish for you is that you will be inspired by the *Three to Be™ Program* and the story of its creation and jump into any part of it that you choose. Transforming your life is not easy! It takes structure, discipline, drive, and dedication, amongst many other things. For me, it all came down to this: I had lain upon the emergency room table way too many times. There are many things I want to do in my time here on Earth, and I didn't want that time to be chock full of struggling because of food anymore. Creating the *Three to Be™ Program* was the lesson that the Universe was trying to teach me so that I would never have to be on

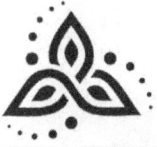

THREE TO BE

Healthy

▼

Step 1

**CHANGING
MINDSET**

Step 2

**FINDING A
NORTH STAR**

Step 3

**BUILDING A
SUPPORT TEAM**

Safe

▼

Step 4

**CREATING A
SAFE-CARE PLAN**

Step 5

**EXPANDING
AWARENESS TO
HEALING**

Step 6

**COOKING
CONSCIOUSLY**

Well

▼

Step 7

**LEARNING
TO ADVOCATE**

Step 8

**DESIGNING A
FOOD ALLERGY CARD**

Step 9

**HUMANIZING
FOOD ALLERGIES**

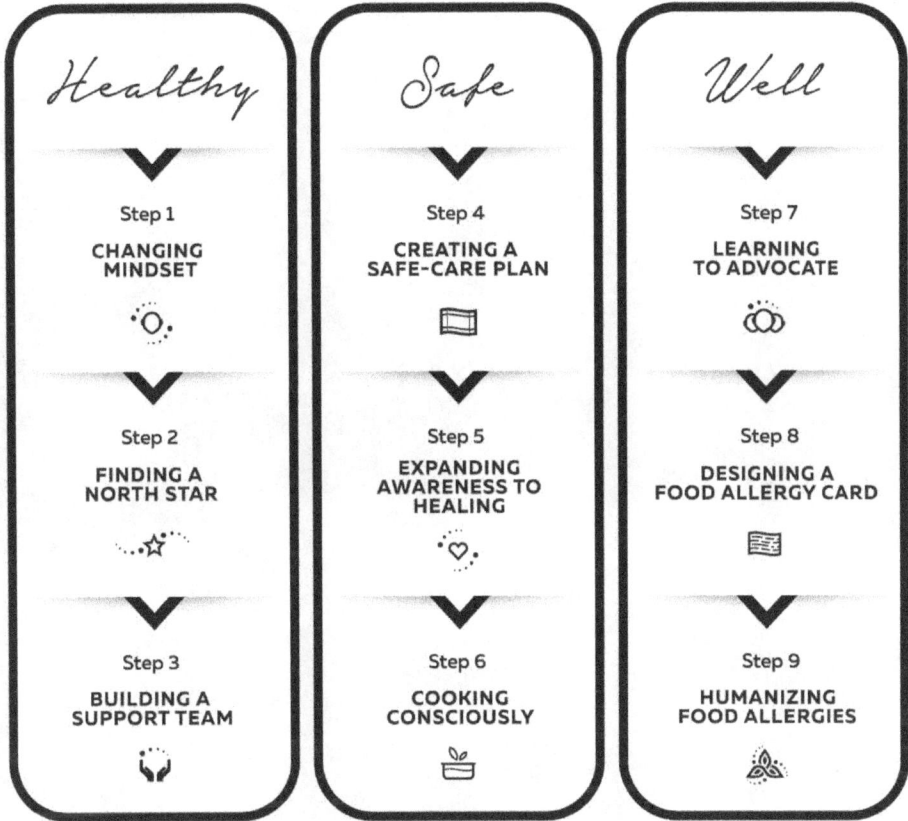

that ER table again. The lesson was all about doing things differently than I had done them *before* in order to really live *now*.

Just as I wanted to see myself *Be Healthy, Be Safe + Be Well*™, I truly wish this for all of you who are on your own personal journeys to well-being. I want you to be free to experience all of the beauty life offers to us, and I want to empower you to manage your food allergies so that you are able to do exactly that.

PART 2

Be Healthy

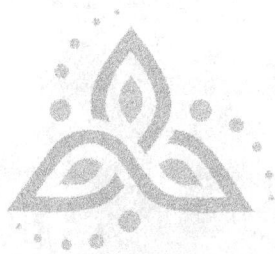

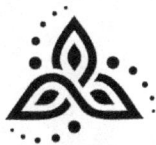

THREE TO BE

Healthy

Step 1

CHANGING MINDSET

Step 2

FINDING A NORTH STAR

Step 3

BUILDING A SUPPORT TEAM

Safe

Step 4

CREATING A SAFE-CARE PLAN

Step 5

EXPANDING AWARENESS TO HEALING

Step 6

COOKING CONSCIOUSLY

Well

Step 7

LEARNING TO ADVOCATE

Step 8

DESIGNING A FOOD ALLERGY CARD

Step 9

HUMANIZING FOOD ALLERGIES

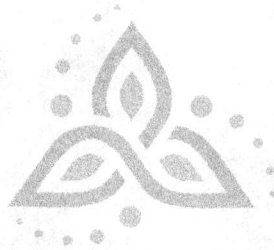

It took almost dying for the fourth time to make me realize that being healthy was about more than just getting rid of my food allergies—I had to incorporate emotional, spiritual, and mental health into whatever I did. Over the year that I had hives all over my body, I began a quest to redefine everything related to my health and well-being. This new journey of transformation began with asking myself the question of "How do *I* define being healthy?"

The World Health Organization (WHO) defines health as "...a state of complete physical, mental and social well-being and not merely the absence of disease or infirmity".[20] When having discussions with friends on what being healthy meant to them, the answers I got varied: "I feel healthy when I'm not carrying extra weight on me" and "I feel healthy when I'm not sick" and "I feel healthy when I'm not stressed out." Another friend told me that "not having an illness doesn't necessarily mean you are the epitome of health. Being healthy means something different to all of us, because we deal with different things." She was absolutely right.

Health and wellness is a personal journey for each of us. Focusing only on my physical health from my initial diagnosis until my adult years led me to struggle with my mind, spirit, and emotions, all of which affected my overall health. But physical health only represents *one* element of an individual's total health! There are actually four areas of one's overall well-being:

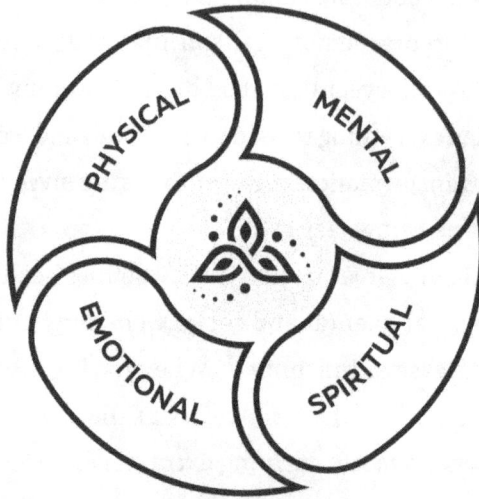

- **Physical** health refers to the state of our physical body and how well it's operating.

- **Mental** health refers to our cognitive, behavioral, and emotional well-being. It is about how we think, feel, and behave.

- **Spiritual** health is achieved when we feel at peace with life. It is when we are able to find hope and comfort even in the hardest of times. It is important to note that spirituality is different for everyone.

- **Emotional** health means that we are aware of our emotions and have control of our thoughts, feelings, and behaviors.

These four areas together define holistic health. I had not been taking care of my health from a holistic perspective, so I began journaling once more to define what all of this meant to me.

Being healthy meant that I could be active, recover quickly, and age gracefully without having to take a million pills a day for various illnesses. I wanted my body to be in shape, I wanted my mind to be strong, and I wanted to live a joyous life filled with love. To get more granular, being healthy also meant:

- Embracing my health situation.

- No longer having disease.

- Not having any more anaphylaxis attacks.

- Not having any more hives.

- Being able to eat a variety of foods that didn't make me sick.

- Being able to quickly recover from ailments.

- Aging without additional diseases or other health-related issues.

- Being able to exercise without ailments as I aged.

- Maintaining an ideal weight.

- Having healthy skin, eyes, and hair.

- Having low stress.

- Having peace of mind.

- Enjoying stable and sound mental health.

- Having deep laughter, joy, and love in my heart and in life.

· Feeling comfortable in my own skin.

· Being proud of who I am.

· Loving myself.

And my list went on. It is important to note that when I wrote down "no longer having disease," I was alluding not only to my food allergies and asthma but also to any other potential diseases I could be susceptible to. Although I was going to do everything in my power to hit my North Star, genetics played a big part in why I had food allergies to begin with, and those same genetics would likely play a role in whatever else might come in the future.

Embracing my food allergies would allow me to not always be down about them. In discussions with my doctors, I had realized that the level of my allergies could go from being very severe to being mild—which would be an incredible win! Therefore, being healthy had to first come with embracing the good, the bad, and the ugly of food allergies. With acceptance, I could move forward with new ways to manage any ailments and work toward my North Star. With this in mind, I began thinking about goals for being healthy in each of these areas: body, mind, spirit, and emotions.

In 2008, I was living a goal-oriented life when it came to both work and play. In my tech work life, I am literally measured by hitting goals within a certain amount of time. If they are not hit for some reason, it can be seen as a big failure even though a million other factors I have no control over might be at play. This is true for many people working in tech—for example, if someone doesn't hit their sales goals for a quarter, the feedback from management is focused around what that person didn't do and how they need to improve. Never mind that the entire industry could be shifting! Just think about how many industries had to shift during the pandemic.

I might not have been able to change corporate culture overnight, but I could surely change how I did things in my own life by looking at themes rather than goals—after all, being goal-oriented around my food allergies could lead to failure if I couldn't get rid of my hives or food allergies by a prescribed date. In 2008, I had expected my hives would disappear before I was released from the hospital. Then I kept pushing that date out another week, then another week, then a month. In the process, I became depressed that my goal wasn't happening, and that was all because of expectations.

In reading entrepreneur and best-selling author James Altucher's works, I found a blog post about his ideas regarding living by themes rather than goals. It was written by Niklas Göke. As Altucher sees it, Göke writes, "...your overall satisfaction with life isn't determined by singular events; instead, the average of how you feel at the end of each day is what counts." A goal, he says, is about asking "What do I want?" whereas a theme asks "Who am I?"[21] Altucher's themes are ideals, ones that he uses to charge his decisions; these themes are standards he can hold all of his actions against. Prior to 2008, I was not actively working to try to get rid of my food allergies—I was just suppressing them with heavy Western medications so that they wouldn't ruin my day.

Before my 2008 incident, I had kept a long list of life goals. It was kind of like a bucket list. Thereafter, though, I decided to try living my life themes instead and got rid of the list. I had to believe that the total effectiveness of a group of things interacting with one another is different from or greater than their effectiveness in isolation. The themes I strategized about and added to my whiteboard centered on the notion of holistic health; I would embed these themes across my body, mind, spirit, and emotions.

- Love: Doing everything from a place of love.

- Peace: Pausing and taking a breath when life gets stressful.

- Intention: Knowing my priorities and implementing small daily habits.

- Commitment: Believing in what I am doing.

- Intuition: Trusting myself.

- Soul: Connecting to the things I am doing from my core.

- Purpose: Finding what I am passionate about and living that.

- Truth: Seeking knowledge in everything.

- Justice: Knowing what is right and what is wrong.

Just by writing these down on my whiteboard, I felt decades of stress fall off my shoulders. I believed in these themes! The best example of living by themes coming into fruition for me was writing this book. When I first began writing it in 2017, I researched how to write a book. All of the materials spoke about goals and timelines to hit with your editor. But since I had changed my approach to live by themes and not goals, I decided that writing this book would be part of my life's work in helping others to *Be Healthy, Be Safe + Be Well*™. Therefore, it would come together within the right time frame. I was not going to stress myself out by putting hard deadlines on it while working a full-time job. That thinking has allowed me to peacefully create this journey for you.

Over the next three parts of this book, I will walk alongside you as we explore the *Three to Be™ Program* on a journey to help you *Be Healthy, Be Safe + Be Well™*. Our journey begins with "Chapter 4: Changing Mindset," which was the biggest step *I* needed to take in order to transform my health. This chapter is the most crucial of the *Three to Be™ Program* because a healthy mind is the foundation you will build upon to achieve anything in life. It was the hardest for me to go through because I had to come to terms with years of trauma and I had to relearn many things that I didn't necessarily want to relearn.

In "Chapter 5: Finding a North Star," we'll talk about why this step is so important and how to do it. And finally, rounding out Part II is "Chapter 6: Building a Support Team," which talks about what types of support systems you should have in your life, as this transformation is neither done alone nor in a box.

The *Three to Be™ Program* meant I had to completely deconstruct who I was in order to become the unique and loving human I am today. Please know that this program is not meant to be an overnight fix! (Although I so wish it were.) As you read, learn, and begin to take small steps—called microsteps—on your own, you will begin to see small changes. Over time, those small changes will lead to bigger health and wellness changes that will allow you to speak your truth and free yourself. This is *your* transformation, so be open to everything that comes with it, both the joys and the pains.

Enjoy these next three chapters and know that I am sending you light and love in your journey to be healthy!

Stories of Wisdom on Changing Mindset

How does your mindset determine your health and what are the key elements for a healthy mindset?

Robyn O'Brien, Author of *The Unhealthy Truth*, Founder of rePlant Capital

"In the health and wellness space, we get so focused on what we're putting into our bodies—is it organic, non-GMO, vegan, gluten-free, Fair Trade, keto, and so much more? But equally important as what we choose to put into our mouths is the thoughts we put into our minds. We do a great job of teaching people how to clean up their cupboards and fridges, but what about clearing out the junk in our heads? I'd argue that it's impossible to live a healthy lifestyle for any duration unless we clean out both the junk in our kitchens and the junk in our heads! And usually, the stuff in our heads is a harder purge.

So the exercise is really bringing each thought forward, holding it, examining it, and questioning it. Think, "Does this serve me? What am I getting out of this thought process? Is it a pattern? A habit?" And then intentionally choose to either keep it or get rid of it, the same way you'd get rid of the junk in your kitchen! It's an ongoing exercise, and the process is so similar. You choose what you put in your mouth; now choose what you put in your head. Choose what you decide to keep there! Our thoughts can nourish us as much as our food choices can, so consume mindfully!"

FOUR

Changing Mindset

"Nothing ever goes away until it teaches us what we
need to know."

— PEMA CHODRON

LEARNINGS

In this chapter, we'll explore why and how your mindset gives you
the power to improve your health. You'll learn:

- At any age, we can rewire our brains to unlearn and relearn.

- Thriving in life is directly tied to changing our mindset
  around our health and well-being.

- Holding a growth mindset with an ongoing connection to
  positive beliefs, patterns, and habits can help promote better
  well-being.

MY EARLY YEARS

Prior to 2008, I had three anaphylactic incidents that took me to
the emergency room in a dire situation. Yet when they were over and
I was feeling better, I felt like each incident was a one-off and I made
no changes to my lifestyle. If the definition of insanity is repeating the
same thing over and over yet expecting a different result, then I was
well on my way. My pattern was taking advice from my team of doctors
and continuing to take the Western meds they prescribed to suppress

my symptoms. After 2008, though, I took a good hard look at changing everything I was doing with the intent of getting a different result. In order to do that, the first thing I had to change was my mindset, or the way I was viewing everything to begin with.

WHAT IS MINDSET?

Mindset is the established set of attitudes held by a person, their worldview, or their philosophy of life. Think of mindset as the collection of thoughts and beliefs that shape a person's thought habits. Your thought habits affect how you think, what you feel, and what you do. Your mindset impacts how you make sense of the world and how you make sense of yourself. Much of what we are can be caused by our genetics—although our environment shapes the way we think, biological factors account for up to 70% of differences from one person to the next. But at the end of the day, it all pretty much starts and ends in your mind. What you give power to has power over you if you allow it to!

After going through the trauma of a fourth anaphylactic incident in 2008, my body was a disaster, my mind was mush, my spirit was crushed, and my emotions were all over the place. I turned into "Negative Nelly," and I didn't want anyone pitying me or trying to appease me by saying that things were going to be okay.

"Don't worry, it will all be okay!" was a sentiment I'd hear often from friends. "Shut it!" was my response, because I didn't know if things *really* were going to be okay. I needed to wallow in my pain and be left alone, possibly forever. One of my besties told me that I wasn't a victim and so I should not play one. He continued, reminding me that I was alive, out of the hospital, and working on a plan with my doctors about the hives. But if I didn't change my attitude, he told me, perhaps I would make my situation worse than it already was. In my best British accent, I told him to piss off.

I know, I know... That's a terrible thing to say, especially to a bestie. But I couldn't deal with what he was saying, because he was right—I *was* playing the victim, and I couldn't see beyond it. For weeks, he kept persisting, as if to prove some point. "I wasn't there during those other times when you were in the emergency room, but I see what you're going through right now and it's pretty bad!" he said. "You need to get a grip, get your head back in the game, and fix this so it doesn't happen again. Don't play the victim, understand?" OMG, I was going to throw him out a window!

Of course, he made sense. But I loathed the word "victim." Victims were the characters on *Law & Order SVU* who didn't pay attention to the creeper lurking in the dark behind the trash can. Those unaware characters died. Victims were people who were tricked or duped. That wasn't me! In my journal, I wrote in capital letters *"AM I A VICTIM?"* The answer to that was no, because I was still alive. But I had a victim's mentality, which is what my friend was trying to tell me.

WHY CHANGING MY MINDSET WAS CRUCIAL TO HEALING

Life definitely is not fair. Bad shit happens to good people all the time. Many people blame their lack of health, love, success, and happiness on factors that are outside their control. Everyone experiences hardships in life, and those impacts can justifiably have detrimental effects on our mindsets. But as my parents always taught my siblings and me, there are just as many stories in the world of people who grew up in poverty—with just one parent or one leg; people who had no eyes or were homeless—who went on to achieve great things despite their obstacles. Growing up in India, my parents had seen poverty first-hand every single day walking to and from school.

I worked with a therapist who noted that humans have the power to change the trajectory of their lives if they have the appropriate mindset, grit, and perseverance to do so. On the other hand, having a mindset in which you're constantly blaming negative life events on other people or circumstances will hold you back from succeeding.

Aha! Now what my friend had been trying to say to me made sense. And I agreed. Because after all I had been through, I refused to add the word "victim" to my list of issues.

Our brains have evolved to really like certainty, which stems from our basic drive to survive. We have evolved to predict and control circumstances because doing so optimizes our ability to live. When we experience change, our brain can interpret this as a threat or a challenge—which can lead to distress or negative emotions such as feeling anxious, frustrated, and/or stressed out. Thoughts such as "I can't do this!" run through our minds, causing us to feel stuck in the moment and our current situation without a solution in sight.

In 2008, I was stuck. Years of managing my food allergies via a single plan that included heavy medications to suppress my symptoms and believing that I was doing a great job were thrown out the window in a matter of one night. I had completely disregarded the pent-up, deep, negative effects on my mind, spirit, and emotions, and now they were all on the table. It was like my guts were hanging out. Holistic healing was the only way I was going to get through this.

When we experience change as an interesting opportunity to learn or do something new, we're more likely to experience good stress, because our new environmental demands seem to be within our abilities and limits. This was the mindset I was moving toward: not being afraid of leaving the past in the past and overhauling things for a better future.

FIGURING OUT MY MINDSET TYPE

I had an insatiable appetite for learning about different types of mindsets and determining where I was. If I was at the low end of the scale, you'd better believe I had the fire in me to change that! I read two bibles on the topic of mindsets. One was *Mindset: The New Psychology of Success* by Carol S. Dweck, Ph.D., and the other was *The Brain That Changes Itself: Stories of Personal Triumph from the Frontiers of Brain Science* by Norman Doidge, M.D. In my readings, I learned that when we see ourselves as a victim, that places us in a fixed mindset. That in turn means we are likely to give up before even trying anything. For example, people with fixed mindsets have a tendency to stick to what they know, avoid confrontations or challenges, take constructive feedback negatively, and feel that they cannot improve.

The more positive mindset is that of a victor, because wanting to be a victor means you are striving toward a growth mindset. With a growth mindset, people believe that their most basic abilities can be developed through dedication and hard work—brains and talent are just the starting point. This view creates a love of learning and a resilience that is essential for achieving great accomplishments. People with growth mindsets have a tendency to feel that they can accomplish whatever they set their minds to because they are open to and learn from feedback and they have a "Keep trying and never give up!" attitude. With a growth mindset, you are a student of possibility!

And then there's yet another facet to this thinking, namely a false mindset. That's when a person believes that they possess a growth mindset but are in fact unwilling to change and move forward because they believe that doing so won't be effective. This resonated with me in 2008, because I felt defeated. It seemed like nothing I did was working, so why try? My friend and my therapist at the time were key to helping me understand that it was crucial to change the way I looked at my situation in order to achieve my desired outcome.

HOW I BEGAN TO CHANGE MY MINDSET

Changing mindset is a hard commitment and can take an entire lifetime, but I was on the fast track. I convinced myself that if I didn't change, the next time I was in the hospital would probably be my last time there (and on Earth). In order to change what I was doing, I had to change how I viewed everything related to my food allergies and health. Being an analytical person, I wanted to understand more about how and why I was in this place. In my readings, I found mindset coach and guide Kelly Fryer, who wrote an article titled "9 Signs It's Time to Change Your Mindset".[22] In short, she pointed out you need to change when:

1. You see nothing but negatives.
2. You are relentlessly resisting the truth.
3. You have a tendency to blame others.
4. You are passionately worried about everything.
5. Your expectations are stressing you out.
6. You secretly want a pain-free life.
7. You're never satisfied with what you have.
8. It's been a while since you learned something new.
9. You catch yourself living in the past.

I read each of these several times and felt the pain of each in my core. This was so me, and it made me so sad! I evaluated each one to try to get to the core of things.

1. **You see nothing but negatives:** In 2008, this was absolutely true. But this had a long history attached to it when it came to my health, too: I was negative and always down about my food allergies, and I never accepted or embraced them, which was what I needed to do to save my life.

2. **You are relentlessly resisting the truth:** Yes, I ran around like a madwoman in San Francisco trying to disprove my doctor's food allergy diagnosis in 2008. Once again, I did not accept my situation.

3. **You have a tendency to blame others:** Yes! I blamed the server and the restaurant the night I ended up in the emergency room.

4. **You are passionately worried about everything:** Oh, Lord, for sure! All of my life, I was known as the worrier in my family, and it showed all over my face.

5. **Your expectations are stressing you out:** Yes, the fact that I had expectations in general was apparently bad, according to the copious self-help books I read at the time. This was a new area to explore, because my expectation that life could go back to normal after being released from the emergency room never happened, and therefore I went into a downward spiral.

6. **You secretly want a pain-free life:** Of course! Doesn't everyone? I had dealt with my food allergies for three decades, and the pain had manifested across my body, mind, spirit, and emotions.

7. **You're never satisfied with what you have:** In regard to my food allergies, yes, I wasn't satisfied that I didn't have a healthy life like others did. Constantly comparing my health to others had brought so much negative energy into my life and was weighing heavily on me. This was a huge revelation!

8. **It's been a while since you learned something new:** Yes, this was true regarding my health. I had been using the same techniques to manage my health for three decades,

and obviously, those weren't working. I was definitely set on changing this.

9. **You catch yourself living in the past:** I didn't really remember a time when I was healthy, per se, so my living in the past was tied a lot into #8, meaning I was just doing the same old things over and over. And those things were not healing me.

Talking this exercise through with my therapist validated that it was high time for a holistic change. But we are creatures of habit and those habits are ingrained in us. Could I really just change them overnight, or at all? Making change in any part of my life began with looking at my situation holistically and determining what needed to happen (or not happen) in order to achieve my North Star.

But habits are real, yo! They are ingrained in us throughout our entire lives. How hard is it to kick a bad habit? Well, can you really just eat *one* chocolate chip cookie or potato chip? No! Being back on the emergency room table was a result of a bunch of bad habits. But change was imminent.

I had always overanalyzed everything, but now I was putting a stake in the ground and vowing to never be in that situation again. It was a defining moment when I said to myself, "Nope, not going back there again! Only progressing forward." And that's exactly what I did.

✳

Life coach Tony Robbins says, "To effectively communicate, we must realize that we are all different in the way we perceive the world and use this understanding as a guide to our communication with others".[23] He believes that the keys to success include the ability to make new distinctions about how you perceive your world. Tony and a number of highly acclaimed motivational speakers have implemented the art of neuro-linguistic programming (NLP) to train people to reprogram their minds for success. NLP is a behavioral technology, or a set of guiding principles; it's a way of changing someone's thoughts and behaviors to help them achieve their desired outcomes. It relates thoughts, language, and patterns of behavior learned through experience to specific outcomes.

I've worked one-on-one with a few NLP coaches over the years to learn the techniques necessary to unravel the hardwiring of the past and begin to take slow steps (there's those microsteps again!) to learn anew. Again, this is not something that happens overnight, so taking daily microsteps is the best way to make change over time. Years later, I was super excited to attend the six-day "Unleash the Power Within" workshop, which is Tony's path to breakthrough and where I learned these techniques in person.

Tony's practice includes the concept of metaprograms, which are "the key ways that a person processes information. They are powerful internal patterns that help determine how someone forms their internal representations and directs their behavior. Metaprograms are the internal programs we use in deciding what to pay attention to. Humans distort, delete, and generalize information because the conscious mind can only pay attention to so many pieces of information at any given time".[24] Metaprograms tell your brain what to delete. If you're moving toward something, for example, you're deleting the things that would divert you back toward the old habit. To change your metaprograms, all you have to do is become aware of the things you normally delete and begin to focus your attention on them. For me, this was analyzing the negative habits, patterns, and beliefs in my life that didn't serve my health and well-being.

ANALYZING MY HABITS, PATTERNS, AND BELIEFS

It is important to understand the difference between a habit and a pattern. Transformational facilitator Monika Walankiewicz wrote a great article on this subject titled "Are Habits and Patterns One and the Same?"[25] In the graphic below, Walankiewicz describes why habits and patterns are not the same and why "...understand(ing) the difference, so you can learn how to deal with patterned behaviors and experiences, and most importantly release shame and judgment you have placed on yourself for engaging in self-sabotaging habits."

Surface Level: Habits are a behavioral expression of patterns. You can think of them as symptoms.

These are the things you do.

Mid Level: Patterns are an expression of unhealed emotional wounds, unconscious believes, and stories we formed about ourselves and others based on those beliefs. There can be patterns of experiences, thoughts, or emotions developed as a reaction to past threats or traumas.

Base Level: Those believes formed as a result of past hurts, traumas, and painful things that happened to us. (Usually, they are relegated to the subconscious mind.)

It is the causation level.

For example, I analyzed my previous behaviors around dining out and found the following habit + pattern + belief trio:

- **Habit:** Letting someone order for me at a restaurant.

- **Pattern:** Going back to my same life after an allergy incident and not changing anything.

- **Belief:** I am not worthy of a healthy life.

My belief that the Universe purposely picked me to be sick caused me so much trauma! So, the pattern made sense, because if I believed I wasn't worthy, then why try new ways of being healthy when they would never work? The bad habit then ensued—I would just let someone else deal with my food allergies, because *I* couldn't deal with them. I literally was putting my life in someone else's hands even once I was old enough to actually take care of myself.

Like most things, there are two sides to behavioral patterns: good patterns and negative patterns. Using a method that Tony Robbins calls "question burst"[26], I spent several minutes writing down a set of questions that I needed to answer about my behavioral patterns as they affected my body, mind, spirit, and emotions. My list included:

- What are my top three positive habits, patterns, and beliefs?

- What are my top three negative habits, patterns, and beliefs?

- How did I come to each belief?

- How is each positive habit, pattern, and belief helping me thrive in life?

- How is each negative habit, pattern, and belief holding me back in life?

- What is my ideal state for each negative habit, pattern, and belief?

- What would I do differently if I knew that nobody would judge me, both in my health and in my life?

- What activities help me feel most like myself?

- What excuses do I need to stop making?

- Is anyone a bad influence in my life, i.e., someone who brings out a negative habit, pattern, and/or belief?

- What are some past events that have messed with my self-confidence?

For the first time in my life, I was pouring out my soul. The more I got into the weeds of this process, the better; the more I could answer authentically and truthfully, the better idea I would have of the work I had to do in order to change.

I dropped my answers to these questions into a spreadsheet and then began to analyze them, looking for repetitive words and behaviors. Then I highlighted those.

My top three negative patterns were:

1. **Allowing:** Letting someone else drive my life.
2. **Overthinking:** Worrying about everything.

3. **Suppressing:** Subduing food allergy reactions rather than eradicating them.

It felt so yucky to write this on my whiteboard and see it every day—it was as if I had wasted so much time in my life with nothing of substance! And many other patterns revealed themselves, such as being very hard on myself and not speaking up for myself, both of which were big issues when it came to managing my food allergies.

I went a bit deeper into these patterns to reveal two incredibly important pieces of information (along with the help of my therapist):

- I carried a lot of shame because of my food allergies.

- I didn't love myself.

Gosh, I will tell you that writing those two sentences has made me cry many times, because I really used to believe them! Seeing the innermost parts of my life being exposed by simple black ink on white paper was excruciating. Shame is a nasty, ugly beast. None of us should ever have to feel shame for who we are or what we believe. In her killer TED Talk, *Listening to Shame,* author Brené Brown states, "If you put shame in a petri dish, it needs three ingredients to grow exponentially: secrecy, silence, and judgment. If you put the same amount of shame in the petri dish and douse it with empathy, it can't survive".[27]

The heartbreak in my soul brought on by these realizations made me feel like my life was out of control. Putting all of this on the table was an amazing step toward changing my mindset! I paused there for a few weeks to let everything really sink in. I no longer wanted to feel shame, and I certainly didn't want to not love myself.

CHANGING MINDSET THROUGH MICROSTEPS

The word "microstep" means a small step toward achieving a desired outcome. ("Microstepping" is taking that action.) The inspirational Arianna Huffington, founder of *Huffington Post* and *Thrive Global*, refers to microstepping as the foundation of our behavioral change platform: "By making very small changes, you have the power to change your life. They're small, incremental, science-backed actions we can take that will have both immediate and long-lasting benefits to the way we live our lives".[28]

Just taking one step toward change on a daily basis took the pressure off and kept me from feeling like I needed to overhaul things immediately...and then inevitably feeling depressed when that didn't happen. By addressing and changing my base-level beliefs, patterns, and habits through microsteps, I was changing my mindset.

According to a study from Duke University,[29] around 45% of our everyday actions are made up of habits. Our habits, then, are a fundamental reflection of who we are. In reading this, I felt elated to be on a path of change! I had to work on specific microsteps in order to drive mindset change, and those came with much reflection, contemplation, and discussions with close friends and my medical team. (I came to think of these people as my support team who would accompany me on my journey.) I identified several related areas that contributed to harmful or negative mindsets and identified the microsteps I needed to take to change them.

Harmful Mindset: I Carried Shame about My Food Allergies

A Belief I Had to Change: I had always felt that there was something shameful about having food allergies. Shame arises from a core belief that we are simply not good enough, and for most of my life,

I had felt singled out from the crowd because of my disease. It made sense that my natural reaction was to hide it. To overcome this sense of shame, I worked through the following things.

Step One: Having Self-Compassion. I came to an understanding that having food allergies wasn't my fault. Reading, researching, and having conversations with different doctors helped me gain a deeper insight of the role that genetics and our environment play in our health. Only from that place could I see how much more was involved with my food allergies and that none of it was something that I had done or *hadn't* done. That's when I started to become compassionate with myself.

Step Two: Saying Positive Affirmations. I wrote down anything positive I could think of about having food allergies. For example, I wrote, "You have two eyes, two arms, and two legs." I wasn't kidding. I also wrote, "There is an enormous amount of food you can eat while many people still go hungry every day." That one still sticks with me. I began each day with daily affirmations and even wrote some on yellow sticky notes to place throughout my home.

Step Three: Addressing Fears. I put my fears on the table and started meeting with my besties to talk to them about how I had always felt ashamed of having food allergies and was working to move past that. In therapy terms, this is called "untangling what I'm feeling," and it was the first step to eventually finding my voice and honoring myself. My friends were deeply touched that I would be "so real and true to myself," as a few put it. This was a loving and safe place for me to start addressing fears. Later in life, I would do this on a grander scale and also with people I didn't know.

Harmful Mindset: I Allowed Others to Lead

A Belief I Had to Change: Others were more experienced with my food allergies and health than I was, so I had assumed they should take the lead. To overcome this, I worked through the following things.

Step One: Opening My Mind. I vastly increased my daily reading on topics ranging from mental health to self-help, and I scoured many psychology books to understand mindset better. Then I kept a list of questions that I needed health care practitioners to help me answer as we discussed the steps I was taking to change my mindset around my food allergies. I made it a habit to read two chapters before I went to bed every night and did not veer from this schedule no matter how tired I was.

Step Two: Being Intentional. This was a process of "owning my shit" and doing things with intention going forward. I become intentional about the kind of people and information I let come into my food allergy experiences so that I wouldn't revert back to negative ways. People who were truly supportive would allow me to lead in my own way and with my own style rather than constantly telling me what to do. I stepped this up with my doctors by doing a ton of research on testing and alternative therapies before I met with them. That way, I was able to have a two-way conversation, during which I was able to push their thinking on conventional therapies. It's important to note that this was not me refuting science, rather it was me trying to understand the science at a deeper level. This was me becoming empowered.

Step Three: Creating Boundaries. I set healthy boundaries with *all* of the people in my life (especially the ones I was closest to) by being assertive with what I wanted and didn't want. A big part of doing this was learning how to effectively communicate. Because we all hear and learn things differently, the verbiage I used in communicating my needs was paramount. Taking the emotion out of my communication while keeping the empathy in, I created a list of words that were unempowering and replaced them with positive words. For example, changing "Could you?" to "Will you?"

Harmful Mindset: I Was Letting Life Happen to Me

A Belief I Had to Change: My life was reactive, not proactive. To overcome this, I worked through the following things:

Step One: Taking Responsibility. Sitting my ass in the emergency room bed, I came to the realization that first and foremost, *I* was responsible for myself and my actions. I had to stop blaming everything else for what was happening with my health. Once I started working to change my mindset, I focused on changing my verbiage from "because *they*..." or "*he/she* did..." to "because *I*..." and "*I* did..." I kept catching myself if I fell backward. For example, in training my dog, I've used a clicker, a tool that makes a clicking noise and can be repeatedly associated with a treat or reward. The clicker becomes a conditioned reinforcer. I used this on myself and became very cognizant of the way I spoke. If I found myself going down the "he said/she said" route, an internal "click" would go off in my head and I would immediately stop. This is very hard to do until you get the hang of it, but if you work on this daily, you will almost instantly see positive changes for the long run.

Step Two: Working Through Anger. Anger and shame can be closely tied together. When someone is struggling with feelings of shame, they may lash out at others in anger, as I did with my bestie when he was trying to talk to me about victim mentality. My step here was to journal these feelings immediately as they came up in order to get to the root of them and understand the emotion behind the anger. (My therapist helped with this, too.) I literally would open my phone and dictate a note to myself if I didn't have a journal with me. That repeated behavior created an awareness of the anger and allowed me to own my part in what I was blaming. Again, a click would go off in my head and I would pay great attention to my verbiage and feelings and set an intention to stop placing blame on others. Instead of placing external blame, I would work through what I was feeling with the help of those who loved and supported me. Then I began to verbalize what I was feeling.

Step Three: Acknowledging that Failure is Good. One of the things that holds us back from taking the initiative is a fear of making mistakes. But the opposite is true—making mistakes and failing is a necessary part of growth. I sat down and wrote out a list of every time I felt I had failed or made a mistake and analyzed each one from a perspective of "How did I grow from it?" It was a long list of mistakes! I had to shift my mindset to know that even if I failed with this trans-formation, much growth would come from it. In my journal, I created a table with one column for the mistake and another for the growth that came with it. By making this mindset shift and seeing how much growth had already happened thanks to past failures, I was able to truly embrace being proactive.

Harmful Mindset: I Needed to Know Exactly What Was Going to Happen in the Future

A Belief I Had to Change: I had to control every aspect of my life. To overcome this, I worked through the following things:

Step One: Identifying My Triggers. The first step in being able to let go of controlling everything was to identify what triggered my need to control things. Smart, huh? Uncertainty is a part of life, and I wrote this in big letters across my whiteboard. Constantly bringing up a "What if?" scenario was an attempt to introduce some certainty into an unknown situation. But now I was working to get rid of the worrywart in me, because I was also getting worry lines on my face! In adopting a more mindful approach to build tolerance for uncertainty, I began jotting down what had triggered me into a worry spiral so that I could experiment with methods that prevented me from going down it. For me, getting rid of thinking in terms of "What if?" related to my allergies was huge! The minute my mind went to a "What if?" I clicked it away and started the thought over again.

Step Two: Being in the Moment. We get so caught up in the rat race that the next thing we know, 50 years have whizzed by. Did we really live? And did we live passionately? Personally, I was living in either the past I was miserable about or in a future I was uncertain about, both of which caused me great anxiety and stress. But I realized that the reality of my situation was that I could not predict my future health state. I could only work hard toward having a healthy and happy life and the ability to deal with things as they come. So, I prioritized what I *could* control and worked on daily steps to invigorate a healthy body, mind, spirit, and set of emotions. I began participating in small things that made my soul happy and expanded my mind, such as testing out recipes, reading books in new genres, and hanging out at art museums. My theme was about enjoying life in the moment. This daily "me time," as I referred to it, replenished my soul.

Step Three: Accepting Things. The faster I could move toward what was bothering me rather than denying or running away from it, the faster I could free myself from the pain of needing to control it. So, I began doing a mental dump of my feelings and/or a mindful review at the end of the day in my journal. I thought back to how my day had gone and to any particular moments or events, reviewing how they had made me feel and how they had affected my mood. The point of this was to see the day's events for what they were and positively accept that I had gotten through them.

> **IDENTIFY THE NEGATIVE BELIEF, PATTERN, AND/OR HABIT; REFLECT ON IT; FIND THE ROOT CAUSE; ERADICATE IT—THIS WAS THE PLAN I WORKED ON DAILY TO CHANGE MY MINDSET.**

In this work, I saw things about myself that I didn't like and wanted to change, and I also identified many incredible pieces of who I am that make me a unique individual. No more victim, only victor!

Before I left the emergency room back in 2008, I had whispered under my breath "Never again!" I wholeheartedly meant it. That same fire was still raging inside of me and driving me to do all of this. There was no option to go back to my old ways. The only choice was to choose *me* and to work on beliefs, patterns, and habits that were keeping me from thriving. The only choice was to move forward.

HOW YOU CAN GET STARTED WITH MINDSET CHANGE

This is one of the hardest, yet most life-fulfilling exercises you'll go through to transform your life with food allergies because of all the trauma and drama that goes with them. So, take your time! Don't put timelines on this. Mainly, just be open to whatever happens.

Step One: Put a Stake in the Ground.

- In your journal, write a sentence saying that you have made a decision to change your mindset. You can say, "I will change my mindset of how I view my life with food allergies and my overall health."

- Look at it afterward, then close your eyes. Put a mental stake in the ground to change your mindset around your health and well-being.

- Look at it every day and let it seep in.

Step Two: Define Your Growth Mindset.

- Write down your definition of a growth mindset.

- Create a list of negative beliefs, patterns, and habits that are affecting your health.

- Ideate and write down ideas about how you could change each of your negative beliefs, patterns, and habits.

- Look at all the new ideas you've come up with and feel great about them!

Step Three: Notice Your Thoughts and Reframe Everything.
I used a handful of strategies from the NeuroLeadership Institute[30] that will may help you get started on your growth mindset journey:

- Try reframing your thinking to view change as a challenge, not a threat.

- Celebrate moments of progress during the change, including baby steps.

- Give yourself permission to start experimenting along the way.

- Learn from peers who seem to model the growth mindset well.

- Look for ways to lead by example, even if you aren't always confident.

THE NET NET

Changing my mindset was the single most important step in my transformation, because it opened my mind to possibility. It took being at the lowest of lows to get me to realize that I must do things differently. Because I was at my true rock bottom, I fast-paced this process over a few years, and like an amoeba, I soaked up everything—and in the process, I spat out all of my previous life habits, thoughts and behaviors, and patterns that no longer served me. But I'll repeat: your path is personalized to *you,* so don't put any pressure on this. Once I knew that the path I was on was a much better one, I could take daily microsteps to get to a better place. With these steps (and probably for the first time in my life), I started taking the weight of decades of trauma off of my shoulders, allowing me to feel hope for a long and healthy future. My head began to feel lighter and at peace, and I began to love myself.

Whether we perceive significant moments in our lives as being threats or opportunities alters our physical, mental, emotional, and spiritual experiences. Consequently, it's possible to shift how we experience these change moments through our mindsets. This is not an easy process, because we're unraveling every part of our lives: the good, the bad, and the downright ugly. It's like trying to un-Google yourself—that could take a lifetime! This process is about pinpointing learned behaviors and environmental factors that are negative and then relearning a better way.

I still work on this every day. When I catch myself going into an old pattern, I "click" myself immediately to stop. In changing to a growth mindset, not only was I able to transform my health, I was able to cut out negative patterns, and that also transformed my life. I know the ramifications of past negative behaviors and don't need to ever end up on another emergency room table to be taught that lesson. Over the years of having a changed mindset, I have become open to a world of hope and acquired a set of tools that I need to thrive in life.

So, where do we go from here? Living life based upon the expectations of others is no way to live. And clearly with my ass lying on the emergency room table again in 2008, I wasn't making anyone proud. I had no sense of direction in life, and I didn't know, at the root level, what was and was not important—in my health or in my life. I was floating through life, in a sense. Working on mindset change, I felt the need to make sense of my time here on Earth. This meant figuring out my purpose in my food allergies because they were a part of me.

Now, with my mind finally set on a positive and new path toward better health and well-being overall, my work was just beginning. This desire to thrive in life was way bigger than just a mindset shift! It needed vision, strategy, creativity, and execution. But I was missing one key part: purpose. Once I realized that lack, I sought to find it.

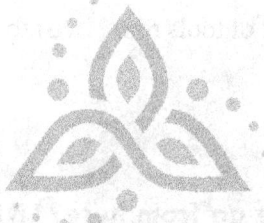

Stories of Wisdom on Finding a North Star

What is the North Star that led you to found the Food Equality Initiative, and how has it guided your life in food advocacy?

Emily Brown, Founder and Chief Executive Officer of the Food Equality Initiative

"I have always been a very civically engaged person. As a teenager, I visited nursing homes to sing and spend time with the residents; in college, I tutored at-risk students. So when food allergies and hunger became a part of my everyday life, I looked for a way to make a positive impact in my community.

When my daughter was a year old, she had an anaphylactic reaction to peanut butter. Thereafter, we learned she was allergic to peanuts, eggs, dairy, wheat, and soy. We immediately had to make many changes to her diet.

My husband and I quickly became overwhelmed with the cost of allergy-free foods and decided to get assistance from the Women, Infant & Children (WIC) program to help feed our daughter. But our daughter was unable to eat many of the foods offered by WIC due to her allergies. We sought assistance at local food pantries, but again, my daughter's allergies prevented her from taking full advantage of the foods the pantry offered.

I realized that there was no safety net for low-income people diagnosed with food allergies or celiac disease, so I created a North Star to become an advocate for individuals facing food insecurity and managing a medically necessary diet. Eventually, I created the Food Equality Initiative."

FIVE

Finding a North Star

"The important thing is to tell yourself a life story in which you, the hero, are primarily a problem solver rather than a helpless victim. This is well within your power, whatever fate might have dealt you."

— MARTHA BECK

LEARNINGS

In this chapter, we'll explore why reflecting on what makes life worthwhile will benefit your health and happiness. You'll learn:

- A North Star can be the theme for your life.

- It can guide you as a beacon of hope and purpose, a true calling in life.

- It will show you just how unique you are in the Universe.

MY EARLY YEARS

For most of my life, spirituality meant participating in cultural events that my Indian parents made us go to. My parents are not religious people, but they did celebrate big holidays on the Hindu calendar such as the birthday of an Indian god or Diwali, our Festival of Lights. Let's get this straight: these events were nothing more than a massive excuse to party. When we were teenagers, my parents would drag us to different events in honor of Lord Ganesha, one of the best-known, and most worshipped of Hindu deities. He is well-known in Western culture as the patron of writers, travelers, students, commerce, and new projects, for Lord Ganesha removes obstacles from one's path. He is widely celebrated in India and other Buddhist communities and recognized by his elephant head and human body. Once a year, my family would attend a celebration in his honor at an event hall that was part of a local church's property. The event was about giving thanks to Lord Ganesha and receiving his blessings, except that my mom had all these annoying rules:

1. We had to wear Indian clothing.
2. We had to eat the vegetarian food that was provided and could not throw any of it away, as it was blessed by Lord Ganesha.
3. We had to behave and act properly.

"Why does Ganesha care if I ate a burger on his birthday?" was my question to mom. She told me to be quiet.

A Hindu priest (or Guru-ji) would conduct a ceremony similar to a Catholic mass service while our parents recited words and sang songs in our Marathi language. All of us kids would mimic the words and faces of the adults as we taunted each other during the ceremony. Then at the end of the ceremony, each family would go up and offer fruit in the tabernacle-like area where the statues of the gods were, close their eyes, and ask for blessings.

"Did you both ask for some smarts and strength? Did you pray for your upcoming SAT score? Don't forget to pray for a good husband in your future," was my mother's commentary to my sister and me afterwards. And once that was all done, the food, drinks, and party began. This is what I equated spirituality with.

Now, although I would not have admitted it then, the solace I received from sitting quietly and having a one-on-one conversation with a Heavenly being was something I thoroughly enjoyed. As a rebellious teenager, I didn't want my mom to get wind of this. But as I grew up, I started to realize how much life can be enhanced by receiving blessings and great juju from anyone who is willing to give them! I may not have talked to anyone about my health situation growing up, but the woman or man upstairs has certainly had an earful throughout my life.

At my mom's encouragement, months after my anaphylactic incident in 2008, I visited a local Hindu temple near San Francisco. "Go and sit there and find some peace," she said. "Don't forget to take fruit and coins with you as an offering for blessings...but not bananas since you are allergic!" She ended her advice with, "Just go and be at peace." Peace was something nonexistent in my life that year.

This particular Hindu temple I visited was quite simple and empty when I arrived. I sat down on the 1950's style carpeted floor, staring at the gorgeous statues of various Hindu deities whose stories I had read in comic books as a child. I saw Rama, the embodiment of chivalry and virtue; Sita, the divine heavenly goddess and wife of Lord Rama; and Lakshmi, the goddess of wealth.

Then I saw Lord Ganesha, and my eyes fixed on the adorned statue of the Elephant God. My eyes narrowed. In my mind, I began asking him why my obstacles had not yet been removed. What had I ever done in my lifetime that was so bad that he would put me through almost dying yet again and make me continue to have hives all over my body? Why, why, *why*? That question started bumping louder and louder in my head until I lost it and started crying. As if he had heard my tears hitting the carpet, the priest came out from the kitchen and sat by me.

"What troubles you, my child? Why are you crying?" he asked.

Uh, hello? Did he not see Jabba the Hutt right in front of him? "Just look at me—I'm hideous!" I said. I didn't have the strength to even look him in the eyes. I was fixated on Lord Ganesha and why my obstacles (in my case, hives) had not been removed.

The Guru-ji asked what was on my skin and what had happened. That led into a longer conversation about how I felt like God either hated or cursed me because he or she kept putting me through horrible allergy incidents in my life. "I must have done something bad in a previous life to have earned this scarlet letter all over my body," I blubbered.

He had a calm and peaceful way about him, the Guru-ji, as he proceeded to tell me that I had not done anything bad in a past life. "I sense you have so much worry, child. This is not good. Always look to God. Don't stop praying or talking to him," he counseled me. "This will all go away. Look within and open your mind, your heart, and your soul to allow the light to guide you. It is within you. Then will you be able to see what is happening here and free yourself."

What the hell was he talking about? His words made me wail even more. What light? Again with the lesson? He was speaking in Hindi, so perhaps my translation of what he was saying wasn't as good as I thought it was. He ended his sermon with, "Be at peace. Be in harmony. Just be."

Although he left me feeling more confused than ever, somehow the Guru-ji's calming words and demeanor did allow me to have my first peaceful night of sleep since I had left the hospital. For weeks thereafter, I prayed every night for the Heavens to show me the light at the end of the tunnel. I talked to a friend who was very into spirituality, and she explained that the word "light" in general reminds us of many pleasant feelings: radiance, brightness, warmth, delight, floating, effortlessness, uplifting, and clarity.

Right now, I was in a place of darkness and devoid of those feelings, but I could turn it all around just by changing the way I viewed things, by focusing on the bright side of life. There was that lesson of changing my mindset again! Now that I was embarking on a journey toward doing things differently as they related to my health, she added that I could benefit from having a mission or purpose guide me down my path. And that purpose would become my North Star.

THE SIGNIFICANCE OF A NORTH STAR

The North Star, a.k.a. Polaris, provided nighttime guidance to slaves escaping to northern states and Canada before the end of the Civil War. Due to its powerful history as a navigation tool—it doesn't appear to move around in the sky the way other stars do—the North Star has become a symbol of the metaphorical beacon that guides our personal growth. The term is also used to refer to a personal mission statement. "When you find your North Star, you know where you're headed. That alone feels good. Plus, your North Star is (presumably) wholesome and vital, so aiming toward it will bring more and more happiness and benefit to yourself and others. And you can dream bigger dreams and take more chances in life since if you lose your way, you've got a beacon to home in on",[31] says the amazing Rick Hanson, Ph.D.

When I was a kid, I used to walk outside, look up at the sky, and recite the children's rhyme "Star Light, Star Bright." Then I would choose the brightest star I could find and make a big wish for the future. The next time I would go out at night, I felt as if that one star was always there, following me and only me throughout my life. It made me feel safe and loved and as if I had some higher purpose. Likewise, you can think of the act of finding your North Star as finding your life's purpose.

Prior to 2008, I had never sat down and defined a life purpose. Why would I? I mean, it's not like they emphasized it in school or at university. When I moved to San Francisco, my purpose was all about being independent and making a lot of money, which I came to realize is not a true purpose. The notion of having a light guide me in a new journey toward holistic health was incredibly important during a time when I badly needed hope. As everything was falling apart, I needed to be able to go outside and find my North Star and feel it, even if for just a few moments. It was almost like a way to reset myself if I was going backward into bad beliefs, patterns, and/or habits. But now I had to figure out what my mission statement actually was.

DISCOVERING MY NORTH STAR

I began this process by reading a book called *Finding Your Own North Star: Claiming the Life You Were Meant to Live* by Martha Beck. "When Dante went off looking for a situation where he could experience the ultimate realization of these qualities, he called the goal Paradise. You can call it Heaven, Nirvana, the Garden of Allah, Enlightenment, a condition resulting from high levels of serotonin in the brain, or Disneyland—I really don't care, so as long as we have some shorthand label for the ultimate manifestation of our potential for good and happiness. I think of this condition as the North Star",[32] Beck writes. Just as explorers depended on Polaris when there was no other landmark in sight, Beck states that "...the same relationship exists between you and your right life, the ultimate realization of your potential for happiness".[33]

Whoa. That last sentence gave me shivers! I too wanted to realize my potential and live the life I was intended to live, just as I want for every single person on this Earth.

Finding my North Star was not easy—it took a long time of

strategizing, writing statements, and throwing those statements out and starting all over again. I didn't need validation from others, per se, but I did run early statements by selected people to see if what I was trying to convey made sense. In the process of doing so, I realized that no one I had spoken with had written down a North Star statement of their own.

This process required much focus and dreaming. I was looking to create a statement that moved me and lit a fire under my ass every time I looked at it. It was bigger than writing down a goal you are certain you will reach—this was about dreaming big! This was about legacy! Here's how I went about it:

Step One: Calm the F*ck Down! Ha! You like my first step, huh? I realized that I needed to calm down, like ASAP. My mind was full of past traumas and future fears, and I could not find purpose if I did not calm my mind. You know that T-shirt slogan that starts with "Keep Calm"? Well, I needed one of those for every day of the week. I was distracted by hives and the 30-plus pills I was taking each day, and sometimes I fixated on that. But the work I outlined in Chapter 4: Changing Mindset started me on the process of becoming calmer, and the ability to calm my being allowed me to focus on change.

To calm my mind, I did two things: I stargazed, and I gave myself time-ins instead of time-outs. Psychoanalyst Carl Jung once said, "If you put yourself into the icon, the icon will speak to you."[34] In other words, connecting with the North Star visually and viscerally can stimulate emotional insight. In a similar vein, San-Francisco based licensed marriage and family therapist Jessica 'Chiara' Viscomi says that "...spending time under the stars has been shown to be beneficial for your sleep-wake rhythms and psychological well-being. Also, experiencing the state of awe while looking at something as vast as the night sky can pique your sense of curiosity, increase feelings of generosity and goodwill toward others, and decrease stress".[35] There was not a night that I missed my stargazing time! (Which was very easy not to miss seeing as I was a dog owner and could let my pup out before bedtime.) It was like making a wish and then sleeping peacefully on it.

The next thing I did to calm my mind was a bit different from the child's version of a time-out. That traditionally involves going to a solitary place, but whenever I felt anxiety and my heart began to race, my time-*in* involved sitting in a sunny, warm spot in my house, closing my eyes, and taking my pulse until it was in a slower, more normal state.

Oh, and thirdly, I added a yellow sticky note to my bathroom mirror that said, "GURL, YOU'D BETTER CALM THE F*CK DOWN!!!" Yes, with three exclamation points.

Step Two: Start Visualizing. Visualization is creating a mental image of having or doing whatever it is that you want. It is the process of picturing yourself with your goal as if it were already completed. To find my North Star, this process began with journaling what my ideal health looked like, being as detailed and descriptive as possible. When my thoughts were calm, I could think through things freely and creatively.

Visualization is always done in the present tense, pretending that something has just happened or is happening now. Using all five senses enhances the feeling that what's being imagined is real so that the mind truly believes it *is* real. I began by building a vision board: I clipped images from magazines and pasted them into a collage that represented the ideal state of health and well-being I was trying to achieve. Those images included physical bodies I was inspired by that came in all shapes and sizes; images of people with bright smiles, laughing and joyous; images of spiritual beings from different religions; and many different representations of love.

I envisioned the following things in detail when I closed my eyes:

- My body is in its ideal state of health.

- My physical surroundings when I achieve this.

- What I am doing in my life and who I am doing it with.

- My perfect daily routine.

- My mind, spirit, and emotions also being in their ideal state of health.

- Role models for this ideal state of health and specific things about those people that make me feel that they could be role models for me.

- Aging gracefully and in good health.

- All of the hardships I've endured disappearing; in their place, a gorgeous light is leading me down a path to achieving my North Star.

- Myself in the state where I achieve my North Star.

I visualized all of this in my mind's eye, and it made me feel joyful and kept my inner fire going to see everything through. Visualization is something I did on a daily basis without fail, as doing so also calmed my mind and allowed me to focus on the bigger picture.

Step Three: Write My North Star Statement. Now the hard work began of writing this damn thing! As a master multitasker, eliminating distractions was the name of the game in order for me to write my North Star. That also meant not putting pressure on myself to get it done ASAP. It was a process, one in which I would need to write it, sit on it and let it sink in, and then finalize it.

As someone who lives and dies by her calendar—both at work and at play—I began time-boxing. I bought a timer, set it, and would begin my task. Once the timer went off, I had to stop and go on to something else. Otherwise, the process was going to be like me working on a presentation and checking Facebook three times per minute on the side.

I turned off my Wi-Fi, calmed down, went into the moment, and focused on the visualizations. If I needed more time, I would just set up another session and time-box it. This process (which I still use to this day) allowed me to focus, and once I was done, I actually felt accomplished.

The North Star statement I created was:

To age healthily by ridding myself of my food allergies."

I am so very proud of the work I did to come to that statement! It resonates with me on so many levels. Getting rid of my food allergies is absolutely a guiding light, but I also accept that it may never happen. If I am able to reduce the severity of my allergies from off-the-charts to mild, then I have already won (as my doctor had pointed out). Even more importantly, I want to be a beacon of hope to others going through their own struggles. I want to inspire and empower them to think differently about their situations. I want to help them live the life they want to live. My North Star was never really just about me—it was about connecting with humanity.

Step Four: Manifesting. Angelina Lombardo, author of *The Spiritual Entrepreneur: Quantum Leap Into Your Next Level of Impact and Abundance*, says, "Manifesting is making everything you want to feel and experience a reality...via your thoughts, actions, beliefs, *and* emotions".[36]

Manifestation began with me believing both in what I had visualized *and* in my North Star. The old me would have stressed out, wondering if that would or could ever happen. But the new me and my changed mindset slapped the silly out of that girl every time she went backward. To really make sure I wouldn't slide, I added a sticky note to my bathroom mirror that said, "STOP repeating the past!"

Manifesting meant being very clear on what I wanted, beginning to ask for it, and starting to work toward it. I knew in my heart of hearts that I deserved everything on my mood boards and then some! I knew I was on this path for myself as well as for others. I knew God had given me so much strength to get through horrible life-and-death situations and keep me going. So, manifesting was all about me taking action toward my newly created North Star on a daily basis. As I did so, I also reconciled myself with the concept that while I might not get everything I wanted, "...having gratitude for what you [I] did have/get is the key," according to Lombardo. True, dat!

Once I had my statement written on my whiteboard, when I would go outside at night to wish upon my star, I would repeat my North Star statement and put it into the Universe, knowing that I was on the journey I was destined to take.

HOW YOU CAN FIND YOUR NORTH STAR

Finding your North Star can be a fun and life-changing experience. You can even create one for your personal life and one for your work life and then align them around a greater purpose.

Step One: Go Deep Within and Strategize. To begin figuring out your North Star, get your body and mind into a peaceful and calm state. Then, as you're in that state, think about these questions pertaining to your life and health:

- What do you love to do?

- What do you want to do?

- What do you dream about achieving?

- What activities set your soul on fire?

- How do you define being healthy?

- What is your ideal state of health?

- What is your ideal state of living?

- Who do you want to be?

- What specific areas of your health do you want to improve?

- What are your deal-breakers when it comes to your health?

- Describe the best scenario for your health and wellness.

- Describe the worst scenario for your health and wellness.

- Describe your top five negative health habits.

- In what ways can you better your overall wellness?

- What things in life make you joyful and exuberant?

- What do you want to share with the world?

- What is your "why" behind each of the above questions?

Step Two: Visualize it in Your World. Move on to the visual-ization exercise and create your visual mood board. As you do so, use these questions as guiding principles. When you begin writing your

North Star statement, take a lot of time to iterate it. Feel free to run it by family members and close friends to get their reactions, *not* their opinions. (I repeat: *not* their opinions!) The more you iterate, the more your creative juices will flow, whisking you along until you get to the statement that just feels right to you. Remember, *yours* is the only opinion that matters throughout this process.

Step Three: Let it Be. Once you've got a North Star statement that feels right, let it be for one to two weeks. Don't touch it. You can look at it, but don't change it. Just let it soak in, and let it be. Your North Star statement should be something you feel proud of, and something you feel is achievable, because it's about to become the theme for your life and you are going to manifest it every day!

THE NET NET

I never want anyone to hit rock bottom, as society has equated that with something negative. But if I hadn't hit my rock bottom, I would never have transformed my life, and if I hadn't done that, I believe I would have died. Novelist Fyodor Dostoyevsky wrote, "The mystery of human existence lies not in just staying alive, but in finding something to live for".[37] For a long time, I was not living—I was existing. And that existence with its many hardships was purposeless. Almost dying yet again showed me that I had to find purpose in why all of this was happening in the first place.

I realized that the lesson that kept repeating itself was me being in the hospital because of my food allergies. But now I was in control of stopping the madness and had a North Star lighting my way! Before 2008, I was not open to or ready for any of this. I am so grateful that one fateful night changed me in a positive way. In finding my North Star, I got to write down all of the things that make me unique in this world—something I had never realized before.

Finding your North Star may seem like a daunting task at first but spending even five minutes a day thinking about it and journaling or whiteboarding about it is a huge step toward transformation. Just making the statement and accompanying commitment to yourself that you are going to *do this* is a step toward your transformation. That said, taking action is what it's all about! Those actions can start off as small daily microsteps that allow you to see progress. Once you get the hang of it, those microsteps will become second nature in your routine. Yes, it takes time to focus, visualize, and manifest. But those are key tools to build in your arsenal, tools that can transform your health and get you through life in general.

So, where do we go from here? If writing the past two chapters showed me anything, it's that I couldn't lock myself in a room for a day and expect to come out with all the answers—everything in life takes patience, time, iteration, and feedback. Likewise, you don't want to be transforming your life within a black box. Rather, feedback can come from a myriad of people in your life, from family to close friends to the doctors who work with you on your food allergies.

Why do I want feedback on something related to my personal health? Because I don't have all the answers! And because I was looking to be inspired by others who had figured out what worked for them regarding their own health and wellness. It really does take a village... And in opening up to others about my struggles, I also learned about theirs, which was eye-opening. Diverse perspectives are the key to life! So, my natural next step was to create a support team who would stand by me as I worked to achieve my North Star.

Stories of Wisdom on Building a Support Team

In what ways have others supported your child (and your family) in living with food allergies, and what has that meant to you?

Sarah Krahenbuhl, Vice President of Social Responsibility and Executive Director of Phoenix Suns Charities at Phoenix Suns

"My son was eight months old when he had his first life-threatening reaction to food. After the allergist's diagnosis, I found myself sobbing in the grocery story as I tried to find safe foods for him to eat. I had no idea where to start, no idea how to read labels past the calories, and no one in my network to help.

So, I did what any other sensible person would do: I turned to social media. There, I was welcomed into a food allergy group that was full of suggestions, recommendations, and explanations. Those families became my mentors and my saviors. They offered recipes, safe brands, and the understanding of things like 'cross-contamination' and 'signs of anaphylaxis.' I truly believe that without those people, my son would be on a feeding tube. But he isn't! In fact, he is a thriving five-year-old who now has lots of safe foods."

SIX

Building a Support Team

"Vulnerability is the birthplace of love, belonging, joy, courage, empathy, and creativity."

— BRENÉ BROWN

LEARNINGS

In this chapter, we'll explore why it's critical to thoughtfully curate people to support you in your transformation. You'll learn:

- A support team is like having a personal board of directors for your life.

- They are invested in your health outcomes.

- They allow you to be vulnerable and help you better advocate for your health.

MY EARLY YEARS

With the advent of online dating, a world of nut jobs have emerged hiding who they really are behind computer screens. Dating back when I was a teenager with food allergies meant only one thing: my parents were on a need-to-know basis! That trend continued into my early dating years in San Francisco, which was probably a good idea since I seemed to attract emotionally unavailable men who were projects. (Just wait for my next book...)

There was a guy I'd often see at neighborhood bars who always eyed me like I was a scoop of his fave ice cream. One day a bold friend of mine took it upon herself to walk up to him and say, "You know, a picture is worth a thousand words, so snap it or go talk to her!" You gotta love your girlfriends.

Fast-forward to my saying yes to a first date with a tall, dark, super-hot Italian stallion named Rodney, or—as the girls and I referred to him—Hot Rod. Hot Rod had been trying to woo me for a long time, but he was more of the shy-and-quiet type. Eventually, though, he found some courage and asked me out.

Hot Rod planned to take me out to dinner and asked if I liked Italian. LOL, an Italian wanting to eat Italian, why the hell not? Italian food was delicious and easy to deal with since I didn't have issues with gluten and could stick to something simple like pasta with olive oil and butter if the restaurant didn't have anything else that was okay for my food allergies. See, I was prepared!

At this point, Hot Rod knew nothing about my food allergies. My plan was *not* to tell him, because I needed him to like me before I could tell him about all of my freakish qualities. I was impressed with his choice of restaurant—it was a trendy new place I hadn't been to yet. He began by asking what I preferred and then chose a rather pricey bottle of white Burgundy. It was as if he had just finished reading a book detailing smooth moves for a first date. My mind was already set on my dinner before we walked into the restaurant: I was going to have spaghetti and meatballs, as I am rather obsessed with meatballs.

When I opened the menu, though, I realized we weren't in Kansas anymore. The restaurant had a prix fixe menu of elaborately named dishes and only two pasta courses, neither of which were spaghetti and meatballs. There were Italian words throughout the menu that I had never seen in my life, all beautifully printed on the linen card-stock menu.

An internal panic set in as I realized I might have to tell the server about my food allergies. I sooo didn't want to go through that in front of Hot Rod! I hadn't thought about looking at their menu beforehand because I expected there to only be a list of pastas and sauces as options. So, I excused myself and ran to the ladies' room, scurrying as fast I could in 3 ½" heels. I locked myself into the last bathroom stall and hit the speed dial.

"Yo! Wait—why are you calling?" my bestie asked.

"I'm dying! I need help," I said.

"You're dying? Should I call 911? Wait, aren't you supposed to be on a date with Hot Rod? Did he stand you up?"

"No, I'm at the restaurant. I'm in the last stall of the ladies' room," I told her.

"Gurl, what the hell are you doing in there? You don't sound like you're dying. Did you kiss him yet? I need the deets," she pleaded.

"No. He brought me to this amazing place that's so gorgeous and we had drinks at the bar, and then...and..." I started to get upset.

"What did he have? Does he drink beer? I can see him drinking a beer."

"What? No, focus! He had a gin martini," I replied.

Simultaneously, we both said "Eww!" because we knew the only way to drink a martini is with vodka, shaken and not stirred, and filthy dirty.

"Okay, so I don't see any problems here," she stated.

My heart was racing so fast that I blurted the rest of the words like vomit. "The problem is that he brought me to the fancy restaurant you and I have been wanting to go to—the one that has the prix fixe menu and all," I blurted.

"And that is a problem why?" she asked annoyingly.

"Because there's no spaghetti and meatballs on the menu and there's a bunch of other stuff that might be nuts and that means I gotta tell him and the server about my food allergies and he's gonna think I'm a freak and that I eat like a six-year-old," I said in one fell swoop.

Silence. "Oh," she said in response.

Girlfriends to the rescue yet again! This one literally talked me out of running out the back door of the restaurant and all the way home. Instead, she told me to woman up and be honest with him. And if he didn't like me after that, then screw him. She quickly built up my confidence and told me to go back and tell the server about my food allergies. "Deal with it, gurl!" was her finishing line.

And so I did, but perhaps not in the way I had envisioned. I came back and started to vomit a bunch of information all over the server about my food allergies and said I didn't understand what was on the menu, yada yada yada. It was as if the music in the restaurant came to a screeching halt as everyone turned around to stare at me. Hot Rod's face went from McDreamy to McDreadful as he and the server said "Holy shit" in unison. My brown skin turned beet red as the server feverishly tried to write down everything I was saying, asking me a million questions and mumbling something in Italian that I'm sure included, "Who let this bitch in here?"

The server told me he was not sure what to do but would speak with the chef. I quietly said thanks and gulped down half a glass of expensive white Burgundy. And then the punchline came.

"Oh, damn, you're so high-maintenance! If I would have known..." And he babbled on.

My face turned fifty more shades of red from the proverbial slap in the face he had just given me. I had never felt so low in front of a guy I barely knew; I was fighting back every tear that was about to pour all over the beautiful hardwood floor. I quickly texted my bestie under the table, and within ten minutes, I was out the door and in her car. Ciao bello, un-hot Rod!

A few days later, after talking it over with my friend, I was glad to have gone through that experience. Hot Rod was definitely not the kind of guy I should have ever dated—how he would support me in life if he couldn't deal with a simple nut allergy?? (Yes, I had us married off in my head before we went on the date.) And he never even apologized when I saw him around the neighborhood again. Whatevs!

Let's fast-forward a few years after that ill-fated date to when I was dating my then-boyfriend, Sebastian. One summer, we took a beach trip with his best friend and his family, which was a big deal for me. Sebastian was enthralled by me—he thought I was the best thing since sliced bread. Because I had known him for years before our friendship turned romantic, he actually knew about my food allergies, and they didn't faze him a bit. In fact, he thought they were something that made me special and unique. Bless his heart!

One night after having drinks at sunset, we sat down for a dinner party on the beach at a gorgeous rectangular table beautifully decorated with candles, flowers, and seafood galore: lobster, steamers, corn on the cob, a slew of side dishes, and a case of wine from Napa Valley (the last was thanks to me). In between bites, I noticed Sebastian eating some food and then leaving the table—only to come back a few minutes later smelling like peppermint. After the third time, I leaned over to find out what the heck he was doing.

"Hey, what are you doing?" Are you diving into the dessert? You smell like peppermint," I said.

"You are beautiful AND smart, Soni! I was brushing my teeth," he said.

"Aren't we supposed to do that after dinner?" I asked.

"Yes, but I was brushing as hard as I could so that you wouldn't get sick from anything I eat," was his sweet reply.

Tears formed in my eyes. "Yes, but silly man, there's nothing here I'm allergic to," I said. "We already checked."

"I just want to be sure so that I can kiss you," he replied.

I had never felt so loved in my life.

I wondered whether Hot Rod would have reacted differently if he had known about my allergies. Perhaps I didn't feel comfortable confiding in him because I was still in hiding about my allergies. Both of these stories—and the countless other dating stories that happened in the years in between—helped me realize that I will always need people to support me and help me watch over my health.

My immediate and extended family were always going to support me, and so were my doctors, but this was about more than just them. After my 2008 incident, I had a real need for mental, emotional, and spiritual support. And all of that needed to come from a team made up of a diverse set of people who loved me and were invested in me. They would become my "ride or die crew," as Vin Diesel so eloquently put it in the *Fast and Furious* movies.

And so, I set off to find my crew and bring them into my world. It's important to note that this process was not all about me—I also wanted to give back to people who loved and supported me in any way I could. I wanted to give them priority and reciprocity in my life just as I knew they would give to me if I were ever in another emergent situation. My former neighbor and close friend, Jenny, who saved my life back in 2008—was a great example of someone who was on my support team. She was invested in me, as I was invested in her. And that is what creating a support team is all about.

THE IMPORTANCE OF A SUPPORT TEAM

Years of hiding my food allergies made it seem like I knew everything about them, but that couldn't have been further from the truth. I'll repeat: it takes a village. Although I was in a constant state of reading and researching, making sense of that information had to be a two-way conversation with my doctors to keep me informed and prepared. The flip side was that at times the information about my health was hard to swallow and I needed love and empathy from others who knew me. That's where having a support team came in.

There are several reasons why having support from others is important. Having support:

- Gives you a sense of belonging.

- Improves your ability to cope with stressful situations.

- Enhances your self-esteem.

- Promotes healthy lifestyle behaviors.

- Reduces stress.

- Lowers blood pressure and other cardiovascular risks.

- Promotes good mental health.

- Alleviates the effects of emotional distress.

It's true that people want to feel independent and like they are always in control, but in creating a support team, we place ourselves in a position to give *and* to receive because we are all in this game called life together.

Think of a support team as having a personal board of directors for your life. According to Harvard Business Review,[38] "In most companies, boards of directors serve as a source of advice and counsel, offer some sort of discipline value, and act in crisis situations..." Similarly, in this step of the process, I was carefully crafting a support team to act in this respect, a team that would allow me to talk things out, a team I could approach when I was dealing with difficult situations or decisions, and a team who would give me the support I needed to get through challenges because they were invested in me.

In business, every person who sits on a board of directors is in some way, shape, or form invested in that business and its positive outcomes. Likewise, a support team is made up of people who can help us look at things in ways that we normally can't because we're too close to the situation. This group can be as big or small as you need it to be, but I cannot stress how critical it is that you think long and hard about who these people are, because you will be both giving and receiving support from them.

In the process of building a support team, I allowed myself to be vulnerable and share what I was going through with my food allergies. With a changed mindset, I learned that finding people (and not just family) who allow you a space to feel comfortable, vulnerable, and able to share—and who won't judge you—is the essence of what I was looking for. I wanted unconditional love across the board, and in return, I wanted to give that back.

BEING VULNERABLE WITH OTHERS

"Vulnerability" was not a word I grew up with; I doubt my parents had learned that word while growing up in India. With so much on their plate regarding my food allergies, adding long conversations about my feelings to the mix wasn't something I felt comfortable doing. Our culture also warned against airing feelings and/or dirty laundry, especially with anyone outside the immediate family. But with a changed mindset, I realized that my food allergies were nothing to be ashamed of. And that's all I needed to break free.

I felt I could expand my support team to include people who touched my life in different ways. Again, the goal here was not to shut people out—rather, I wanted to carefully select who would be part of my team. After my anaphylactic incident, my heart was warmed by calls, texts, emails, and in-person visits from friends, family, and friends of friends who had heard I was in the hospital. "If you need anything, please let me know!" was the repeated message from all. I began to believe that even people who didn't know me well would come to my assistance if I needed it. I believed in the good in people, and I had faith that if I opened up about what I was going through, people would want to listen.

Brené Brown is an expert in vulnerability. I've watched her TED Talk, *The Power of Vulnerability*, like a million times, and I've read all of her books. I especially loved *Daring Greatly: How the Courage to Be Vulnerable Transforms the Way We Live, Love, Parent, and Lead*. Brené defines vulnerability as "uncertainty, risk, and emotional exposure".[39] It's that unstable feeling we get when we step out of our comfort zone or do something that forces us to loosen control. Making the decision to completely overhaul your life because you think you've been doing it all wrong definitely makes you feel exposed and out of control! And it can make you start second-guessing every decision you've ever made.

Brown also states, "When we think of times that we have felt vulnerable or emotionally exposed, we are actually recalling times of great courage".[40] What she means here is that vulnerability used to be thought of as a sign of weakness, but that is in fact *not* the case. It takes being vulnerable in order to make great change in your life. Taking small steps toward that will help you get comfortable with vulnerability. One of those steps is to let go of the constant worry of what other people think about you. And you need to realize that everyone has struggles and is focused on their own shit, not yours. This was big stuff for me to realize!!

After my 2008 incident, I needed the help of others more than I could have imagined, especially since my parents lived on the East Coast. I needed rides to the doctor, market runs to pick up food, and simple conversations when I felt down. With a changed mindset, I realized I had to choose to be vulnerable and speak up when I needed help.

The most important thing I learned in my research was that vulnerability can be leveraged.

LEVERAGING VULNERABILITY MEANS NOT LETTING YOUR FEARS PREVENT YOU FROM MOVING TOWARD WHAT YOU WANT IN LIFE.

This meant I had to be willing to put myself in uncomfortable situations and have uncomfortable conversations in order to learn and grow. That used to make me feel yucky because I felt exposed. But now, I was going to take a chance on it and bring people into my world.

BUILDING MY SUPPORT TEAM

My ex-boyfriend Sebastian was exactly the type of person I wanted on my support team—not only did he allow me to be my authentic self, but he went one step further by protecting me and helping keep me safe. I began to seek out more people like Sebastian in order to diversify my team. (I didn't only want my doctors on my team.) And I also wanted people on my team who had gone through similar health issues so that we could collaborate; I wanted to find people who were emotionally intelligent and spiritually aware and led their lives with purpose. I wanted to meet people who were invested in service to others, because through the process of finding my North Star, I knew I was invested in helping others, too.

In my journal, I put together three categories for my support team:

Core Members: This list included my parents, siblings, and my team of doctors and other healthcare practitioners. This set of people would work on my physical and mental health issues. From my family, the help I needed was to begin discussions about how my food allergies had taken a toll in all other areas of my life. I was pleasantly surprised at how open my parents were to hear me out without adding their opinions. Being vulnerable changed my relationship with my parents, as I began to also see them as friends.

Chosen Members: Family is given; friends are chosen. In creating this group, it was extremely important that I thought about who would be there for me through thick and thin. I knew I had to choose wisely! I chose people from my ride or die crew, some extended family members I was very close to, and even a few chef friends. This set of people would help me with emotional and spiritual guidance, physical exercise, and two-way conversations about dining with food allergies. I kept this group small—about four or five people max—and slowly began to open up about my struggles outside of just food allergies, having conversations about how traumatic events such as being rushed off to an emergency room in the middle of the night made me feel and what I was trying to cope with. I also began discussing backup plans with them to be listed as my emergency contacts in San Francisco. This was the group of people who I'd dine out with often and who would make sure that nobody at the table ate nuts because they didn't want to take a chance with my health. This was exactly the kind of support I needed.

Honorary Members: These were people who had been through major health and/or life transformations themselves, people I could learn from and be inspired by. I may or may not have known any of them firsthand, but as I joined different types of offline and online communities on social media platforms like Facebook, I found individuals who had gone through traumatic health situations and transformed, just like I was doing. With these people, I was able to discuss health and wellness topics, learn from them, and ask for advice. Through online influencers, I was able to read personal stories of transformation that were publicly shared in news articles, interviews, and podcasts. I wanted to model what these people were doing to transform their lives. By reading their stories and interacting with them on social media, I was able to get tidbits that resonated with me. This information had a dramatic and positive effect on my mind and gave me courage to begin to share information about myself with others.

Now, I didn't go around and tell people, "Hey, you're now a member of my support team—lucky you!" Rather, I set out to have a conversation and build a relationship with each person. That relationship was not transactional but more authentic and vulnerable, even when it came to my doctors. We discussed everything, from advice on health matters to advice on cooking, dining out, and finding new workouts. The topic of "How did you get the courage to tell your story and then put it on Facebook?" even came up. The conversations were raw and personal and there was a lot of hugging. (Each person I met with literally got to see me in my rawness, because I had hives all over my body.) This was a scary process at first, but because these people showed empathy, sharing got easier and easier as time went on.

BECOMING FULFILLED THROUGH THE SUPPORT OF A TEAM

Having a support team has allowed me to speak my truth. I have learned many things in this process:

- There is no shame in being vulnerable.

- People did not judge me because of my health issues. Instead, they respected me for sharing my deepest struggles.

- I authentically showed up for these people. In return, they authentically showed up for me.

- Specific friends became family because I chose them as such.

- The process of finding the right people allowed me to deal with mental, emotional, and spiritual duress from the past and gave me courage.

HOW YOU CAN BUILD YOUR OWN SUPPORT TEAM

Author Sylvester McNutt III states, "Be mindful, extremely selective, and very intentional about the people you allow in your life".[41] He is so very smart in writing this! Building your support team is not a popularity contest. It is about searching for the right people who give you priority and reciprocity, people who love you and give to you unconditionally—and in return, you reciprocate. We all have a million acquaintances and lots of people we call friends. But when things go wrong, you have to have the right people around. So, I encourage you to dig deep within and find those people who inspire you to be the best version of yourself and keep you going when you are down. You are looking to build trust with these people, which is a biological reaction to the belief that someone has our well-being at heart.

Step One: Create Your Lists. In creating your lists, consider the following:

- What do you want to accomplish with your support teams?

- Draw out different categories/teams of people. You can follow my three categories if you'd like (i.e., Core, Chosen, and Honorary).

- Take time to carefully decide who gives you priority, reciprocity, unconditional support, love, positivity, inspiration, etc. Put their names into each circle. Consider diverse backgrounds and experiences when thinking of these people.

Step Two: Share with Your Peeps! Even if in tiny bits, start a conversation with each person to tell them what you are doing. Allow the vulnerability to flow both ways. It is incredibly connecting to verbalize your commitment to someone; that is the reciprocity you will be giving back to them.

Step Three: Reach Out When You Need Help. No form of support is too small. The point of all of this is to reach out to those people when you need help, so test your process and your people. If they are not cutting it, rethink who else could be part of your team. Your safety and health are the number one priority here, so don't feel bad about swapping people in and out as time goes by and life happens.

THE NET NET

Building a support team is one of the most crucial things you can do for yourself, especially when you have severe food allergies. Doing this will help you realize that you are not maneuvering through life alone, nor should you. As we grow and age, sometimes we feel like relying on others is a limitation, but that is absolutely not true. I would say it is just the opposite—as we grow, we need each other more than ever to get through life's hard punches. The people on your support team will also evolve as you evolve! And just as you are being supported, if you are being authentic to yourself, you will be reciprocating your support to your team members and seeing as this is a two-way street. Remember, vulnerability can be leveraged!

So, where do we go from here? The hardest work I went through to transform my health and well-being was what I laid out in these three chapters of "Part II: Be Healthy." That is because in the process of changing my mindset, I was unraveling every part of me that I had once known and turning it around to learn a new, healthier way of being. I was dedicated to the process, and it took time. To this day, I still work through it.

The three steps of changing my mindset, finding my North Star, and creating my support team were baseline steps I had to complete in order to build a strong foundation for my transformation. Only with a healthy mind could I begin to create a healthy body, a healthy spirit, and healthy emotions. As I took daily microsteps, I continued to look inward and get into the weeds of what I needed to do to ensure I would be healthy in all of those areas. I was determined to be responsible for my own safety.

In the next part of the book, "Part III: Be Safe," I detail three additional steps that saved my life. They revolve around education and acquiring levels of knowledge about my health that I didn't have before. (I used the tools described in "Chapter 4: Changing Mindset" in order to open my mind to new forms of healing.) It's important to note that you don't have to approach your situation the exact same way as I did mine since your journey is personalized to you, but you can draw from my experiences and begin to think about which pieces of what I did might help your situation.

Your body is the *one vessel* you have during your time on this Earth! How much you want to invest in it and commit to it is up to you. Ask yourself what level of investment and commitment you want to give as we wrap up the first part of this journey and enter into the next: "Part III: Be Safe."

PART III

Be Safe

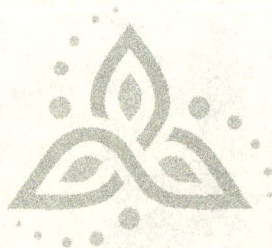

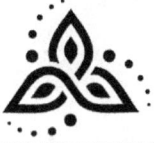

THREE TO BE

Healthy

Step 1
CHANGING MINDSET

Step 2
FINDING A NORTH STAR

Step 3
BUILDING A SUPPORT TEAM

Safe

Step 4
CREATING A SAFE-CARE PLAN

Step 5
EXPANDING AWARENESS TO HEALING

Step 6
COOKING CONSCIOUSLY

Well

Step 7
LEARNING TO ADVOCATE

Step 8
DESIGNING A FOOD ALLERGY CARD

Step 9
HUMANIZING FOOD ALLERGIES

The mantra conversations with my parents that led to the main principles of the *Three to Be™ Program* focused a great deal on safety. As the mother of two girls, mom was always concerned about our physical safety. She had a "strength in numbers" philosophy that she applied to everything: going to/from the school bus stop, walking to the market, visiting friends in the neighborhood. (My sister and I were latchkey kids in the 1980s, so we let ourselves into the house after school and had been told to do our homework and not leave the house. However, that instruction didn't preclude us from running around the corner to pick up a snack without telling my mom.) Similar to my early years, whenever I later thought about "safety," I mostly focused on my physical safety.

As we move into "Part III: "Be Safe," you'll see how I had to learn that safety was about more than just physical safety. It became about my ability to take care of myself safely and healthily. It became about accountability. The realization that I was responsible for my own life was a huge one! So, in being safe, I began to envision what I needed to do to take ownership of my food allergies and manage them in a holistic way that would move me toward my North Star.

I never really knew what the term "self-care" meant until I moved to California and saw people actively taking care of themselves holistically rather than going to the doctor throughout the year. There were actual businesses focused on helping people decompress and reduce stress! I had never seen those kinds of businesses on the East Coast.

The University of Buffalo's School of Social Work defines self-care as "Self-care refers to activities and practices that we can engage in on a regular basis to reduce stress and maintain and enhance our short- and longer-term health and well-being. Self-care is necessary for your effectiveness and success in honoring your professional and personal commitments." They also state that "There are common aims to almost all self-care efforts:

- Taking care of physical and psychological health

- Managing and reducing stress

- Honoring emotional and spiritual needs

- Fostering and sustaining relationships

- Achieving an equilibrium across one's personal, school, and work lives".[42]

In short: it's all related. In order to reduce stress, I first needed to acknowledge that I was indeed stressed. Then I needed to be in the right mindset to *de*stress—which again was something I was actively working on. For example, going for a run helps clear my head when stress comes on. I'm typically running somewhere familiar, with good street lighting, people all around, and not in a bad part of town. Those factors make me feel safe doing that activity and allow me enjoy it, which is what self-care is all about. Another activity I love to do for self-care is getting a deep tissue massage after a long run. I definitely don't want some creeper touching me, so I only go to a reputable and highly recommended salon in a safe location. Being safe allows that self-care activity to be joyful, too. See a theme here?

Any activity I do to take care of myself must start with me being safe—physically, emotionally, mentally, even spiritually. It's not just about just *one* of those, it's about *all* of those together. If we go back to my date with Hot Rod, I was physically safe in the restaurant at dinner, but I was not emotionally safe in general with him; thus, I did not confide in him beforehand about my food allergies.

When I was creating the *Three to Be™ Program,* I thought a lot about self-care as it related to my food allergies. I came up with the concept of "*safe*-care" and wrote that down, because anything I undertook doing for my transformation had to begin with not putting myself in harm's way. I wasn't going to take any unnecessary chances just to write a book. I had to go into every exercise with education, openness, and consciousness.

CONSCIOUS DECISION-MAKING IS WHAT IT MEANS TO BE SAFE IN THE THREE TO BE™ PROGRAM.

In looking at my health holistically, safe-care had to include mental, spiritual, and emotional safety as well. I needed to understand those aspects and how they would allow me to safely manage my food allergies. A lot of what I evaluated in "Chapter 4: Changing Mindset" was focused on the decisions I was making *un*consciously, so I changed my mindset to make them *consciously.*

Physical protection naturally extends to our emotional sense of safety, of feeling secure in a place and within an environment so that we can express ourselves without fear of negative reactions from others. In the next three chapters, beginning with "Chapter 7: Creating a Safe-Care Plan," you'll first learn why I needed to create a safe-care plan to make better, *conscious* health and well-being decisions and how I made that plan. With a changed mindset, I also began to be open to new ways of safely managing my food allergies. That was something I was never open to pre-2008; I detail this process in "Chapter 8: Expanding Awareness to Healing." And finally, in "Chapter 9: Cooking Consciously," you'll see how learning how to cook has literally saved my life many times over.

Incorporating mental, spiritual, and emotional safety into my daily life has allowed me to improve communications, be creative, show courage, and be open to share and learn. I was able to practice all of this because I had created a support team that encouraged me to keep going. And I was able to be vulnerable and speak my truth because I knew what that truth was. It's all related, like gorgeous ingredients in a stew!

Enjoy these next three chapters and know that I am sending you light and love in your journey to be safe!

Stories of Wisdom on Creating a Safe-Care Plan

What does holistic health mean to you, why is it so important, and how do you and your family practice it when dealing with food allergies?

Dina Hawthorne-Silvera, Co-Founder and Vice President of the Elijah-Alavi Foundation

"Because I grew up in a family that had brought their culture to a foreign land, before I knew the term 'holistic,' it was already my lifestyle. I was taught that I am more than just a body. To be holistic is to cater to your total wellness: your mind, body, and spirit.

Living a holistic life is also about finding the balance between the medical model, the Divine, and the Creation all around us. It's about ensuring we are taking care of all parts of us, because the mind, body, and spirit all need each other like blood needs oxygen and the lungs and brain need the heart.

My family and I practice a holistic lifestyle when it comes to our food allergies. We don't just avoid foods that can cause our death—we are also intentional about how mental and spiritual fatigue can manifest or exacerbate physical complications.

Having food allergies can be such an isolating experience within a community of ableist-minded individuals! Not only do you have to worry about food, but there's also a lack of emotional intelligence, and worse, there's a lack of compassion. We believe that our words can break down and build up; therefore, we are careful when talking about ourselves, and we counter negative self-talk with positive declarations. We also lean on our faith and prayer. We are empowering our eight-year-old son with the language and confidence he needs to not walk through life in fear. Our holistic approach will teach him that he is responsible for taking care of his mental and spiritual wellness, because that's not something that can fit into his emergency bag."

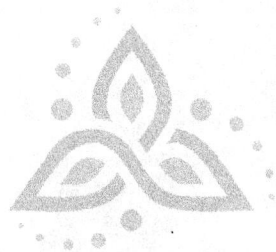

SEVEN

Creating a Safe-Care Plan

"The challenge is not to be perfect—it is to be whole."
— JANE FONDA

LEARNINGS

In this chapter, we'll explore how creating a safe-care plan allows you to prioritize safety in every aspect of your transformation. You'll learn:

- Conscious decision-making is at the heart of a safe-care plan.

- Focusing on food, lifestyle, and environmental changes is necessary for holistic healing.

- Understanding genetic predispositions and gut health will allow you to build a personalized safe-care plan.

MY EARLY YEARS

When I was 13 years old, my mom, younger brother, and I took a trip to visit family in India. One of my mom's sisters and her family live in a small town outside of Mumbai. This sister is unique—she's a rebel, a badass, and the life of the party. I just love her! She's the one who does things without asking for permission and doesn't bother with what others think. My auntie is the epitome of an empowered woman: comfortable in her own skin, oozing with confidence, she takes no shit from anyone. I worshipped these qualities growing up, secretly wishing they would rub off on me as I was more of a wallflower.

When we would visit her home, she would take my sister and me shopping to show off her "foreigner nieces," as if we were china dolls on display. Similar to Kramer from *Seinfeld* fame, she'd wave hello to every person and she'd say "Look at my beautiful nieces!" in our mother tongue as we went from store to store.

Visiting family in India always included copious amounts of eating. Auntie would prepare food for days, cooking all kinds of scrumptious items we loved. During one particular visit, she made shrimp biryani, chicken kabobs, fish curry, lamb chops, and a few Indian vegetables... all in the same meal! Lord have mercy! As tradition goes, whatever was put on our plates was to be eaten.

"Eat as much as you want, because you won't get my great cooking for another few years when you visit again," she would say.

The after-dinner food coma was met with trays of desserts. I usually didn't partake because most Indian sweets are laden with nuts. Seeing that I was not reaching for any, her son proclaimed that he would eat my share *and* his.

"Why are you eating double the ladoos?" my auntie asked her son. "You already ate too much at dinner! You know you are going to be fat like us one day."

"I'm eating Soni's portion," my cousin said. "Because she didn't eat any."

"She doesn't have to eat it—she'll become fat also," my auntie replied.

This statement puzzled me. I mean, why the hell would I become fat if I wasn't eating any sweets? I gave auntie a weird frown, which she immediately noticed.

"Soni, my pretty girl," my auntie said. "Come here. You are built like us, like our side of the family, not like your father's side who are all skinny. We once were skinny too, and then one day...*POW!* Now look at us. Fat and happy."

I almost fell out of my chair, not knowing whether to laugh or cry. I was stunned at hearing this form of reasoning.

She finished with "Here, have at least one ladoo! There is no pistachio, so half the calories."

Everyone in the room laughed as she made her jokes, but some knob viscerally turned from left to right inside my head at that very moment. I stood up from my chair, put my fist in the air, and yelled, "I will never be fat like any of you! Just watch!"

A burst of laughter at my expense came out of everyone.

But I've kept my word all these years later. Look who's laughing now! That was my first lesson in genetic predisposition, only I didn't know it at the time.

UNDERSTANDING GENETIC PREDISPOSITION

Over the past few decades, hypotheses have emerged about how race, ethnicity, and genetics contribute to allergy development and gut health. Research suggests that food allergies emerge from a mix of genetic and environmental influences. Genetic predisposition means that someone has an increased likelihood of developing a particular disease based on their genetic makeup. A genetic predisposition results from specific genetic variations that are often inherited from a parent; therefore, having an in-depth understanding of your family history has a direct effect on your future health and safety.

Children inherit pairs of genes from their parents, getting one set of genes from the father and one set from the mother. Those genes can match up in many ways to make different combinations. Families also share habits, diets, and environments, and those factors influence how healthy we are later in life. Let me tell you, I learned none of this in health class while growing up! I don't believe this is actively taught to kids in school today either, but I feel that it should be as genetic predispositions and family influences have a dramatic effect on how we take care of ourselves in America.

At the end of 2009, when my hives had completely dissipated, my doctors and I began running more allergy tests to determine what was going on. We also began a process of understanding my genetic predispositions. In the Harvard Medical School's article titled "Direct-to-Consumer Genetic Testing Kits," they state, "All disease is, to some degree, genetic. From cancer to the common cold, almost every human malady known to humankind has something to do with genes—the stretches of DNA containing instructions for making the proteins that govern how our bodies are built and how they function. Your genes influence your risk for degenerative disorders—the innumerable conditions from osteoporosis to Alzheimer's disease in which structure, function, or both deteriorate. They also influence allergic reactions, your ability to fend off infection, how you process nutrients and drugs, and even your susceptibility to accidents".[43]

For example, some people are genetically predisposed to developing certain types of cancer. These people have a higher risk of developing the disease than those in the general public. Studies also suggest that while your genes may determine up to 80% of your weight and body shape, environment and personal choice still play a significant role. So, my smart auntie was truly foreshadowing when she said that all of us grandkids would end up like her side of the family partly due to our genes and partly due to choices such always keeping sweets in the house. Therefore, the more I could learn about my family's health history on both sides of the family, the more I could be proactive and keep myself safe from what was to come.

I went straight to the sources that most people go to in order to find out about their genetic predispositions: my parents and the Internet. Okay, of course I also met with my doctors and discussed this, but I had to do my own digging! I researched genetic predisposition deeply and took different over the counter DNA tests such as 23andMe and Ancestry.com, to find out if there something my parents didn't know. I sent in saliva samples and in return was given a report on certain aspects of my genetic health, including:

- Genetic health risk

- Carrier screening

- Wellness and health traits

- Nutrition

- Fitness

- Cellular aging

This was a new way of looking at holistic health that I had not spent time on previously. I was setting out to learn more about my family connections to my food allergies and what else I could possibly be prone to as I aged. And on top of that, if my North Star was to age healthily using mechanisms that were safer for my body, then I also needed to understand what was going on with my gut health.

GUT HEALTH'S RELATIONSHIP WITH FOOD ALLERGIES

I knew diddly squat about my gut health back in 2008, or why I even needed to pay attention to it. The only relationship I had with these words was my gut instinct—that tiny little voice/feeling inside that guided my decisions. According to *Time Magazine*, "...in recent years, scientists have discovered that the gastro-intestinal (GI) system has an even bigger, more complex job than previously appreciated. It's been linked to numerous aspects of health that have seemingly nothing to do with digestion, from immunity to emotional stress to chronic illnesses, including cancer and Type II Diabetes".[44]

It was only in the past five years that I started reading about links between gut bacteria and food allergies in mainstream articles. I learned that each person's gut microbiota is unique but that shared factors and characteristics (diet, age, sex, lifestyle, genetics) influence it. "Microbiota" refers to specific microorganisms that are found within a specific environment. A study by scientists at Vanderbilt University in Nashville, Tennessee that was published in the journal *PLoS Biology*[45] in 2018 found that a person's ethnicity is a better predictor of the microbial community in their gut than other variables such as body mass index (BMI), age, and sex.

If someone has food allergies, when their immune system encounters a food that it perceives to be an allergen, it produces Immunoglobulin E (IgE) antibodies. These antibodies bind to allergens and cause hives, shortness of breath, and anaphylaxis—symptoms that can result in death. These antibodies are the reason why some people swell up when they just sniff nuts while others can eat them without any issues. A 2020 study in *Science Magazine*[46] also pointed to the gut as being the home of these allergy-causing antibodies.

Dr. Cathryn Nagler, Ph.D. and a food allergy professor at the University of Chicago, has been studying the linkage between gut health and food allergies. According to *Scientific American*, "...Nagler and several other researchers are working to find ways to treat food allergies more easily and durably. They're targeting what they believe is a root cause—imbalances in the community of beneficial bacteria, or microbiomes, that lives in our guts—in the hopes of resetting the immune system. ... And in March 2020, scientists reported finding large amounts of antibodies against peanut allergens in the stomach and gut of allergic patients, further supporting the idea that the gastrointestinal tract is a hotspot for food allergy regulation and treatment. Already, companies are testing several strategies".[47]

This was all quite alarming to me, as the state of my gut health was never something I had discussed with any of my doctors as a child or as an adult. I promptly went searching for people who worked in holistic and alternative medicine in online and offline community groups. In our conversations, these people asked me questions like "Have you tested your gut bacteria?" and "Have you been tested for SIBO?" and "What supplements do you take?" and "Do you work with a functional medicine doctor?"

My answer across the board was "No," and regarding supplements... well, I was taking a Women's One A Day daily and that was about it. Functional medicine doctor? I didn't really even know what that was or what that type of doc would do. So, my plan became to continue to research and learn about gut health and its possible connection to food allergies, understand more about functional medicine, and get recommendations for a great partner to work with.

Functional medicine is a personalized and integrative approach to healthcare that involves understanding the prevention, management, and root causes of complex chronic disease. It is practiced by licensed medical professionals and utilizes the most current scientific knowledge regarding how our genetics, environment, and lifestyle interact as a whole system. Once it is understood how that whole system interacts for an individual, then functional medicine professionals diagnose and treat diseases based on patterns of dysfunction and imbalance. Determining the root cause of the illness is an essential component of this branch of medicine.

After years of searching for the right partner, I was lucky to get an intro to Dr. Jill Carnahan, M.D. Along with using functional medicine to help patients find the root cause of their illness, she identifies nutritional and biochemical imbalances that may be contributing to patients' symptoms. I had to kiss a lot of frogs to find my princess in the form of Dr. Jill! She is in high demand and has a very long waiting list, but because I knew gut health was such an important piece to achieving my North Star, I was patient. Upon our first meeting, she immediately connected with my story and North Star and talked of her own parallel health transformation that I could relate to. I was so excited that she got me! I was hoping that by working together, at the least, functional medicine could drastically reduce the severity of my food allergies.

We discussed the ailments I was dealing with and went in-depth on digestive issues. Were digestion and elimination problems at the root cause of my symptoms (and possibly all disease)? Were healthy digestion and elimination the foundation for extraordinary physical, mental, and emotional health and well-being? I was curious to find out with the help of Dr. Jill.

When I imagined my gut as a physical entity, I pictured something that resembled a tube. If the contents within it were toxic and diseased and I just kept adding to its misery...well, of course I was going to be sick, and for a long time. But if we were able to figure out the state of my gut health, and how to get it into an optimal state, then perhaps that would positively affect my food allergies. This was a good theory, and we had much testing to do.

BECOMING A HUMAN TEST CASE

Determined to leave no stone unturned, I embarked upon what often seemed like a million tests, but necessary to get to the information I was seeking. *Your* testing plan should be personalized to you—we'll get to that in the "How You Can Create Your Safe-Care Plan" section of this chapter. For now, just humor me in my insanity. I set out to be a human test case and learn as much as I could through a long list of IgE tests to create a safe-care plan. My testing plan also included some very specific IgG tests, which were new to me in general. IgE is an indication of hypersensitivity or a true allergy, while IgG is a secondary response usually associated with a previous exposure to an antigen. While IgG testing is not FDA evaluated, Genova Diagnostics states, "...An IgG Food Antibody Panel can be ordered as a stand-alone test or bundled with other profiles. Oftentimes, clinicians will bundle several smaller profiles in order to see a more complete picture of the patient's immune-mediated response."[48] Remember, I was leaving no stone unturned, so as much of the picture I could understand, the better. Once the results came in, I discussed them with Dr. Jill, my allergist, and my primary care doctor because they all were a part of my support team. But we relied on the IgE testing results as true food allergies that I needed to watch out for.

- **Genetic Testing:** I had never run these over-the-counter types of tests before, and I was curious. The results from the 23andMe and Ancestry.com DNA tests showed that I was genetically prone to thyroid disease and Type II diabetes (both of which actually ran in my extended family,) age-related macular degeneration (also which ran in my extended family,) and late-onset Alzheimer's disease.

- **Gut Health Testing:** We ran what felt like a gazillion tests in different areas; we did a GI-map; we tested vitamin D and cholesterol levels; we ran IgE food allergy tests and IgG food sensitivity tests, environmental elements tests, mycotoxin tests, mold exposure tests, and even a Lyme disease test. Results at the time showed very high levels of vitamin D, elevated LDL cholesterol, and high levels of arsenic! There were also signs of intestinal permeability, also known as "leaky gut" from the standard lactulose/mannitol permeability assay test, and antigenic permeability screen.

- **Skin Prick Testing:** Results from these IgE tests showed that in addition to my repeat offenders of peanut and all tree nuts, on a scale of 0-4, my results showed new food allergies to: corn (4+), halibut (4+), cantaloupe (3-4), honeydew (3-4), sesame (3-4), and soy (3-4). All of my environmental allergies were off the charts and still at a 4+++ rating.

- **Total IgE Blood Testing**: There are specific IgE classes for these tests ranging from 0 to 6, with a corresponding level of allergen specific IgE antibody from Absent/Undetectable to Very High Level, respectively. Within peanuts and tree nuts I was still in the "Very High Level" category at the time.

- **Pulmonary Function Testing:** Results from the spirometry test (which measures the amount of air the lungs can hold and how forcefully one can empty air from the lungs) showed that my forced vital capacity (FVC) was 63, which meant "moderately abnormal." My forced expiratory volume (FEV1) measured 64, which also was "moderately abnormal."

Waah!! Are you crying like I was? But I remained calm and positive, because the more I knew, the better informed I would be to keep myself safe—and also because I had been working on calming the f*ck down as bad news came in. I gained a deeper level of understanding about IgE and IgG testing during this process. Learning about component level IgE testing was fascinating to me! Keeping myself safe was not a goal, it was now a main theme of my life. In the last ten years, I had found out that gluten intolerance runs in my immediate family, so that was another one to add to the list of genetic predispositions even though my IgE test results showed no allergy to wheat. (Of course, gluten is found in more plants than just wheat.) With all of this under my belt, I set out to devise a safe-care plan that was proactive and holistic, one that would keep me safe from current and potential future harm.

TWEAKING MY SAFE-CARE PLAN WITH CONSCIOUSNESS

I had a lot of information to sift through! For the life of me, I couldn't understand the elevated LDL cholesterol level—I prided myself on cooking at home and eating healthy. Yet this was where genetic predisposition could come into play (again). As a teenager, I remember certain extended family members discussing their high cholesterol levels as they hit their 50's. Which was also the first time those family members purchased gym memberships to 24 Hour Fitness and made immediate changes to their diet. Even though I ate well and exercised daily, now here *I* was with an elevated LDL. It was incredibly frustrating. I felt like I was already trying to make up for how I was (or wasn't) managing my food allergies, and now I had to deal with *other* genetic predispositions that were manifesting in my life?? It felt like for every one step I took forward, I took two steps back. But I kept repeating to myself, "Girl, you got this!" (Yes, that also went on a yellow sticky note.)

I created a safe-care plan built on the theme of conscious decision-making and focused my changes on three main areas: food, lifestyle, and environment. I also knew that if I could continue to be calm, clear, and focused, then I would be disciplined enough to make change.

> **CONSCIOUS DECISION-MAKING MEANT THAT I NEEDED TO FIND MORE MEANING IN THE WAY I WAS GOING TO KEEP MYSELF SAFE IN EACH OF THESE AREAS.**

CHANGING MY FOOD PLAN

Creating a new food plan that was safe for me and holistic in nature meant:

- Removing new allergens from my diet.

- Eliminating foods that were negatively affecting my gut health.

- Making new, conscious decisions about the food I could eat in order to better my overall health.

As I was dealing with new food allergies, high LDL cholesterol, gut health issues directly tied to certain foods, and a genetic predisposition to Type II diabetes, the sources of the food I was eating became paramount. Labels such as "organic," "sustainably produced," "grass-fed," "local," "non-GMO," and "farm-raised" became crucial to my ability to clean up my gut health.

Step One: Cleaning Up My Food. I went through my pantry and refrigerator and got rid of all the obvious new offenders: anything with soy, sesame, or corn, including my beloved microwave popcorn. That was so sad! For months, I also went on a gluten-free diet just to be proactive and to monitor the amount of bread and carbs I was eating. That was very hard given all of my allergies, but it made me focus a lot on vegetables, which made my body feel great! This process required me to use a spreadsheet to keep track of what I could and couldn't eat. Dr. Jill recommended I take my time to adjust to each change in my food plan as she knew I already had so many limitations, but I needed to go cold turkey for months to get into a groove.

Then I began reading the labels of *all* of the not-so-obvious offenders to see if they contained any allergic items such as corn, soy, and/or sesame. Guess what? They did, and a shit ton! Corn is freaking in *everything*! According to The Cornucopia Institute, "Half of the US farms growing corn to sell to the conglomerate, Monsanto, are growing GMO corn".[49] And this: "...genetically modified corn has been linked to health problems, including weight gain and organ disruption." In speaking to my allergist how to go about updating my food plan with the new allergic items, he also had me avoid cornstarch and corn syrup and all other items derived from corn. The plan was to completely eliminate these new allergic items and then retest in six to nine months to see where I was at.

I ran through this same exercise with the other items: halibut, cantaloupe, honeydew, sesame, soy. Halibut was interesting. FAACT, the Food Allergy & Anaphylaxis Connection Team, states, "Allergy to finned fish occurs in roughly 1% of the population and is more common in adults as compared to children. In children with allergy to finned fish, the allergy is typically lifelong. Furthermore, 40-60% of the time the allergy is developed during adulthood, and these individuals are also unlikely to experience resolution of the allergy. Since the allergenic protein (parvalbumin) in finned fish is similar regardless of the type of fish, greater than half of individuals who are allergic to finned fish are allergic to more than one type of fish. Although any type of fish can cause allergy, the most common types implicated in allergy are salmon, tuna, and halibut".[50] Who knew? And why does almost every restaurant in the US have halibut on their menu?

Step Two: Lowering My Bad Cholesterol. High cholesterol increases the risk of heart disease and heart attacks. Medications can help improve cholesterol, but there was NO WAY I was going that route. If anything, I was still working on getting *off* of all the medications I had been on since 2008. In speaking with my primary care doctor, she explained that the main ways I could lower my LDL cholesterol were through diet and exercise. With diet, these were the best ways I could begin to reduce that number:

- **Reducing saturated fats,** which are found primarily in red meat and full-fat dairy products. I completely stopped buying red meat and cheeses, and I looked at alternative milks for my tea.

- **Eliminating trans fats** that are found in vegetable oil, margarine, and sweets like cookies and cakes. I completely stopped buying vegetable oil and began testing out sunflower and safflower oils in my cooking, and also put the kibosh on all sweets (so sad!) for a time period knowing that I may indulge on special events such as my birthday.

- **Eating foods rich in omega-3 fatty acids** such as wild salmon, wild shrimp, and flaxseeds. I stayed true to only wild fishes that were sustainable and avoided darker-meat fishes like tuna, and King Mackerel that contain toxic mercury. I gained a tremendous amount of knowledge about the mercury levels of different fishes during this process.

- **Increasing soluble fiber** from foods such as oatmeal, Brussels sprouts, and apples. Caveat: I also learned that Brussels sprouts contain high levels of arsenic, so I monitored how often I chose that vegetable.

My purging continued. With all of this information, I got rid of the Wesson vegetable oil in my house and went back to my Indian roots and began cooking everything from scratch. The goal here was testing and tweaking to find what worked and what didn't work for my health. I learned how to make homemade ghee (a.k.a. clarified butter) which was a staple ingredient used in Indian cooking. Ghee from grass-fed cows is rich in omega-3 fatty acids and is an important source of fat-soluble vitamins. In addition, ghee has antioxidant properties for your skin and hair. I interspersed ghee, sunflower and safflower oils in my cooking, throwing away the cans of PAM cooking spray. I also switched my breakfast from having nothing to having a bowl of gluten-free oatmeal or steel-cut oats (without any sugar) on some weekdays to begin getting the fiber that I was missing and that I needed to help my gut health. Thank God I wasn't allergic to oats! I made sure to eat vegetables for snacks, and I also made sure veggies were always present on my lunch and dinner plate.

Step Three: Tracking My Food. I tracked every ingredient and dish I ate with app technology, which I still do today. (There's an app for everything...literally!) I tried apps like Lose It, iMapMyRun, Step Track Lite, Lose the Belly, Daily Burn, Fitness Pro, etc. until I settled on Under Armour's My Fitness Pal. I also tracked the ingredients in the foods I was eating. Once you build up your database, it's pretty easy to log foods. Just having my full nutritional information at my fingertips at all times was so insightful!

LIFESTYLE CHANGES

Diversification continued into lifestyle changes as I began to incorporate alternative forms of exercise and movement into my lifestyle in order to improve my cardiovascular and digestive health. Physician, *New York Times* best-selling author, and founder and medical director of The UltraWellness Center Dr. Mark Hyman is one of my all-time favorite people to learn from when it comes to health and wellness. Dr. Hyman suggests that "Exercise and stress can both impact inflammation on a molecular level, through regulatory effects on the immune system. This is a big reason why moving our bodies in different ways can have many amazing whole-body benefits." He continues that "... although we've known that aerobic exercise benefits cardiovascular health, we're now seeing that all types of movement—even slow and mindful practices like yoga and tai chi—additionally benefit our body through decreases in blood pressure, body mass index, and even cholesterol".[51] Once again, I found this information insightful and was excited about trying out new ways to heal.

Step One: Getting the Right Tools. I threw out my Fitbit and upgraded to an Apple Watch, which had more sensors and offered more insights about my health. It was connected to my iPhone's Health app, where I could view detailed information about everything from daily activity levels to body and heart measurements to nutrition and sleep patterns. If there was something to track, Apple was *on* it!

Step Two: Diversifying my Workouts. As the self-proclaimed Queen of Cardio, mixing up my exercise plan was not something I was excited about. A long, fast-paced outdoor run was the only way I felt like I could get a great workout and an adrenaline rush. But I was open to change and incorporating more holistic forms of exercise into my routine.

My dad was a yoga guy, and as children we'd laugh as we watched him curl up like a pretzel in his long johns. He got after me about trying it, especially now. Johns Hopkins Medicine states, "Regular yoga practice may reduce levels of stress and body-wide inflammation, contributing to healthier hearts. Several of the factors contributing to heart disease, including high blood pressure and excess weight, can also be addressed through yoga".[52] With that in mind, I tried many forms of yoga until

I found Vinyasa yoga, where poses are strung together to form one fluid sequence of movements. I also found Restorative yoga, which is ideal for anyone with minor injuries, restricted movements, or lots of stress—and for road-running warriors like me.

I added regular weight-training routines, as it's the only kind of exercise that makes muscles bigger. Bigger muscles generate more strength and especially in women. During this time I discovered the kettlebell, and fell in love! I purchased a set at home, watched hundreds of YouTube videos to establish a great form, and started swinging away to a sculpted and strong body! I had kept up my running, but I incorporated a treadmill run on certain days for less impact on my knees and ankles. I also began running to slow songs, like love songs. I know that sounds funny, but that advice was given to me by a professional athlete, so I was intrigued. He said that he'd been listening to love songs playlists for years during his workouts and in practice. That allowed him to push out the noise and peacefully concentrate on the ball.

At first, I giggled (also because he was so fine) at the thought of listening to "Endless Love" on a five-mile run, but at his insistence, I tried it and became a believer. In the process, I felt myself more connected to the song, the street, and the world I was running by.

Step Three: Incorporating Natural Supplements. For years, I took a daily Women's One A Day multivitamin, probably because someone told me I should. It was no longer cutting it. Now that I was focused on creating healthy gut bacteria and also boosting my immune system, I needed to find a personalized regimen of all-natural supplements with the help of my functional medicine doctor. In addition to vitamins, dietary supplements can contain minerals, herbs or other botanicals, amino acids, enzymes, and many other ingredients that benefit gut health. A simple example of this are probiotics, which were also recommended to me by my primary care doctor. Probiotics are tiny microorganisms that deliver health benefits to their host and are believed to help with digestive issues. Working with my functional medicine doctor on my digestive issues and leaky gut syndrome led to incorporating various herbal supplements personalized for me: gentle and full-spectrum binders containing activated charcoal, gut shield products that support GI barrier health and integrity, magnesium citrate for digestion regulation, ascorbic acid to support the immune system, two different types of probiotics, and a liver essentials product containing milk thistle extract and selenium along with glutathione, omega-3 fatty acids, and some other detoxifying herbs. All of these supplements are made of natural, herbal ingredients and were prescribed specially for me by a medical doctor after analyzing my many test results. Almost immediately, my digestive issues began to be resolved.

Step Four: Detoxing Regularly. I decided to run my own detox program at the beginning of every year for one quarter. The idea was to eliminate any accumulated toxins of various sorts that had built up in my body. Detoxing was about shedding the things that didn't serve me, which included toxic foods, patterns, and lifestyles. For three months every year, I:

- Avoided alcohol

- Avoided sweets

- Avoided white flours

- Did a monthly juice cleanse

- Participated in intermittent fasting three days per week

- Drank one gallon of water daily (yes, one gallon!)

- Had a weekly massage

Step Five: Controlling My Stress. And finally, I had to cut back on the stress in my life, starting with reducing my work travel. My career choice had me traveling all over the globe; during certain years, I traveled 100 percent of the time. Being on the road for weeks at a time is incredibly hard from an eating and exercise perspective—you have to be so disciplined! Regardless of how glamorous the destination was, I made a choice to prioritize my health and limit my work travel to 25 percent maximum per year. This was a dramatic decrease and a decision that my boss at the time was not happy with. But going through a transformation meant not letting someone make me feel guilty about things, especially if I could delegate the trip to someone on my team who could step up! In that situation, everyone wins.

ENVIRONMENTAL CHANGES

Our genetics don't necessarily change that quickly, but our environment can. Our environment can affect human health, and promoting human health can also affect the environment. Environmental hazards increase the risk of cancer, heart disease, asthma, and many other illnesses. These hazards can be physical (i.e., pollution, toxic chemicals, food contaminants) or they can be social (i.e., poor housing conditions, poverty).

It's challenging to pin down exactly what factors cause an environmental health problem. Health problems related to the environment are complex and develop for a variety of reasons, including how prone a person is to develop a disease or condition based on their genes. (Scientists call this "genetic susceptibility.") What we do know is that an environmental health problem is likely linked to physical, biological, and even economic factors. A study by the UC Davis Environmental Health Sciences Center states "The air we breathe, the water we drink, the food we eat and the homes, buildings and neighborhoods we live and work in can all contribute to environmental health problems, sometimes by disrupting how the body works".[53]

This information really touched me. Planetary health was not something I was focused on pre-2008—I never questioned the food print impact I was having on Earth until I myself began to transform. So, I opened my mind and began to deeply understand the impact that our food has on our bodies *and* the planet. I needed to go past just restricting foods I was allergic to!

MY TRANSFORMATION WOULD REQUIRE BEING CONSCIOUS OF EVEN ALLERGEN-FREE FOODS.

"The current global food system requires a new agricultural revolution that is based on sustainable intensification and driven by sustainability and system innovation," according to the EAT-Lancet Commission study. "This would entail at least a 75% reduction of yield gaps on current cropland, radical improvements in fertilizer and water use efficiency, recycling of phosphorus, redistribution of global use of nitrogen and phosphorus, implementing climate mitigation options including changes in crop and feed management, and enhancing biodiversity within agricultural systems. In addition, to achieve negative emissions globally as per the Paris Agreement, the global food system must become a net carbon sink from 2040 and onward".[54]

The data doesn't lie. Researching reports such as this, I was beginning to see the consequences of our food, lifestyle, and environmental choices.

This required me to make immediate change in the following ways.

Step One: Overhauling My Products. I was already remedying what was going *into* my body, but there was another dimension: what I was putting *on* my body. I began throwing away all of my skincare and makeup products in an effort to seek out only products that were certified clean. I researched products that were free from potentially carcinogenic, toxic, and hormone- or endocrine-disrupting ingredients as well as ingredients that have been linked to very serious health issues. I ran through the same exercise with my house cleaning products, detergents, soaps, and anything else in the kitchen that might be toxic to the environment. (Kudos to amazing companies such as The Honest Company and Juice Beauty, and who make clean and nontoxic products we can all feel good about!) The final key product that I switched over to was an all-natural, broad-spectrum toothpaste. I did this because your mouth is the gatekeeper of your gut, and can mirror health and disease in your body. In my research I came to understand that the oral microbiome is a collection of bacteria that affects the progression of health and disease. An imbalance in the oral microbiome can lead to inflammation, illness, and disease. Bacterial populations in your mouth can make their way to the gut bacteria and can alter immune responses, potentially leading to systemic diseases. This information paved a new way of thinking about the ingredients in the toothpaste and mouthwash that I was using.

Step Two: Purifying My Air. Placing an air purifier in the main living areas of my home helped sanitize the air by removing allergens, pollutants, and toxins. Given that I live in California and unfortunately, we have a fire season every year, running these year-round really helped me maintain a safe and clean environment in my house.

Step Three: Researching Plant-Based Foods. Search data from Google Trends shows an impressive worldwide increased interest in veganism starting in 2004. Going vegan was not something I was interested in doing because I already had so many food restrictions, but the up-and-rising plant-based movement was interesting to me from two perspectives: health and the environment. I spent a lot of time researching plant-based diets and how they could benefit someone with food allergies as well as the environment. I'll cover this in more detail in "Chapter 9: Cooking Consciously," but the main step I took was to completely cut out buying red meat. In an article in *The New York Times*, they report that "Cows also put out an enormous amount of methane, causing almost ten percent of anthropogenic greenhouse gas emissions and contributing to climate change".[55] The Meatless Monday campaign, started in 2003 by Sid Lerner, also states that "Eating less meat and more healthy plant-based foods can help reduce the incidence of chronic preventable diseases, preserve precious land and water resources, and combat climate change."[56] So this was my first step toward contributing to a positive food footprint and eating much cleaner to keep myself safe.

HOW YOU CAN CREATE YOUR SAFE-CARE PLAN

According to data in a study in *Science*, "The gut microbiome is environmentally acquired from birth".[57] Therefore, knowing your family history can help reduce your risk of developing health issues in general. Even though you cannot change your genetic makeup, the ability to be *pro*active about your health rather than *re*active is key. An understanding of gut health and genetic predispositions allows someone with food allergies to create a personalized safe-care plan with a theme of conscious and clean eating that also applies to their lifestyle and the environment.

Step One: Learn About Your Genetic Predispositions. Start with the obvious choice: mom and dad! Having a conversation with your parents and/or immediate family members about their health history is crucial to knowing what you could be dealing with in the future. Do some digging, talk to past doctors, and gather any medical records that you can in order to get an accurate picture. If you're like me, you can whiteboard all of this information and see how it connects before discussing it with your doctor and creating a preventative safe-care plan.

At-home genetic tests are also another route. I did that and then took my results to my primary care and functional medicine doctors to get their thoughts before moving forward on anything. There are more than 1,000 genetic tests currently in use, including molecular, chromosomal, and biochemical; more are being developed. So, take the time to work with your doctors to figure out what course of action is appropriate for you.

Step Two: Explore Your Gut Health. Dr. Tara Menon, M.D., states, "In recent years, your gastrointestinal tract has been linked to numerous aspects of health, like emotional stress and chronic illnesses such as cancer and diabetes".[58] We're also starting to see more research on the link between gut health and food allergies. Given all of that, understanding your gut health is one of the most important steps you can take to achieve better health when you have food allergies. In partnership with a functional medicine or naturopathic doctor—who are experts in holistic health practices and herbal treatment options—work on testing to understand your gut's current state and how to improve it. This process can be a great complement or alternative to how you treat your food allergies.

How do you begin to find the right medical professional to work with? Ask your primary care doctor or allergist as they should have a good network of referrals. Also, check out trusted community groups on Facebook or other platforms, and don't be shy about asking for recommendations in the group chat or via direct messages. Asking friends or acquaintances whom you know are really into their health if they know of or work with a holistic practitioner is a more personal avenue to take.

Finally, if you begin gut health testing with your doctor, keep track of your test results in a journal or spreadsheet and utilize mobile apps to track the changes you may ultimately make to your diet and exercise. Review the data you receive and ask your doctor for help with making sense of it all. The insights you will gain will allow you to carefully create a safe-care plan that will lead to positive results.

Step Three: Amend Your Food, Lifestyle, and Environment. It is never a bad decision to review the state of your food, lifestyle, and environment and make changes for the better. Use all or some of my steps in the previous sections to research and think about where you need to adjust. No change is small in any of these areas, whether it be going plant-based, only using all-natural products, and/or going even *more* green to help out the planet. All of these steps will help reduce the toxicity within and around you.

Use journaling or whiteboarding as a part of that process and do so through the lens of consciousness. The more conscious you can be about your food, lifestyle, and environment, the larger impact you can make on your own safety.

THE NET NET

Repeat this to yourself every day: "My body is a temple." After all, it's the only vessel you get while on this Earth, so it should be a priority to make sure it's safe and performing well. When I changed my mindset to look at my whole being this way, I began to seek deeper knowledge about my health and my life with food allergies than I ever had before. I started understanding what works and what doesn't. More importantly,

I started understanding *why*.

Having full disclosure of my situation was central to the decisions I made about my current or future state. Data provided me with the context to create a safe-care plan and then test and tweak that plan in order to achieve my North Star. "Being safe" is an underlying theme in the life of anyone with food allergies: safety within our bodies, minds, spirits, and emotions.

Remember that having food allergies is partly genetic and partly environmental. Gathering good data is not about how many tests you get—rather, it's about working with your healthcare practitioner to choose the most relevant tests from a breadth and depth perspective in order to get a full picture of what's really going on.

You are in control of your results! Don't wait until another food allergy or health issue creeps up that puts you in a reactive state. Doctors can't make us healthy.

WE NEED TO REALIZE THAT OUR GROWTH IS OUR RESPONSIBILITY.

So, where do we go from here? Being able to eradicate my food allergies got down to finding the root cause and effect, and Western medical philosophies are unfortunately not focused on finding root causes. Making changes to my food, lifestyle, and environment would be a huge benefit, no doubt. But I was seeking more. Who else was thinking about food allergies the way I was? What were their methods and techniques? In the next chapter, you'll see my transformation come to a pivotal place as I was forced to expand my mind to other forms of healing to get to my root causes and achieve my North Star once and for all.

Stories of Wisdom on Expanding Awareness to Healing

What role can alternative forms of medicine such as functional medicine play for someone with chronic diseases like food allergies?

Dr. Jill Carnahan, M.D., ABIHM, ABoIM, IFMCP

"I've always been passionate about seeking answers to complex problems. I became a doctor because I believed in the capacity of the human body to heal and overcome even the most dire circumstances—*if* given the right tools. As a survivor of both breast cancer and Crohn's disease, I'm passionate about teaching patients how to live well and thrive in the midst of complex and chronic illnesses. The powerful medications I was given to calm the inflammation in my body from Crohn's disease never addressed my underlying problems. Refusing to believe that surgery and medications were the only options, I made major changes in my own diet, eliminating gluten, dairy, and all processed foods and eating nutrient-dense options instead. A naturopath also taught me the power of appropriate nutritional supplementation in restoring my health and energy and healing the inflammation in my gut.

Functional medicine is no longer considered 'alternative.' It combines the best of conventional allopathic science, genetics, and physiology with additional tools for healing. At the core of food allergies is a hyper-permeable gut. Functional medicine can help restore function by addressing gut permeability with the '5Rs': remove, replace, reinoculate, repair, and rebalance. When applied to various chronic problems, the 5Rs can cause dramatic improvement and sometimes even complete resolution of symptoms. Having utilized this in my own healing, my greatest moments in life are when I see my functional medicine patients—many of whom came to me suffering from complex illnesses that had baffled traditional medicine—transform from a place of despair and pain to a place of resilience, joy, hope, and love."

EIGHT

Expanding Awareness to Healing

"Discomfort is always a necessary part of the process of enlightenment."

— PEARL CLEAGE

LEARNINGS

In this chapter, we'll explore the fact that people living with food allergies are constantly looking for alternative ingredients. Why not also look for alternative ways to heal? You'll learn:

- New, holistic, and empathetic ways to manage food allergies that can help you heal more naturally.

- Scientifically proven options for identifying the underlying cause of disease rather than just prescribing a cure for the symptoms.

- Alternative therapeutic regimens that allow you to address the mind, spirit, and emotional traumas that are related to living with food allergies.

MY EARLY YEARS

When I was in grade school, I became obsessed with eating sandwiches for lunch. Friends brought in their fave sandwiches like tuna fish and PB&J, which I wouldn't dare touch for fear of death. I sought refuge in the world of normal school lunches, where "normal" meant not being sent to school with basmati rice, daal, and Indian snacks.

One day, a friend brought in a bologna and cheese sandwich and offered me a bite. The odd pinkish circular patty underneath fluorescent orange cheese mesmerized me! Without thinking, I took a bite and was hooked. I ran home from school raving about the new sandwich I wanted to eat, but my mother's answer was "No! If you want a sandwich, I will send you to school with a chutney sandwich because it is healthy and has medicinal properties!"

Now, a chutney sandwich is quite delicious—but for an adult, not a second-grader! And "medicinal"? Hmm... Let's start with the fact that it's green in color as it's made with natural ingredients: fresh mint, cilantro leaves, green chilies, freshly shredded coconut, fresh lemon juice, a little water, and salt. You blend it into a paste and put it on buttered bread along with some thinly sliced cucumber. My mom was probably not thinking that showing up to school with a green sandwich that resembled mold would be an issue, but then again, she never went to grade school in America.

The next time we went to the market, she picked up the bologna package, read the ingredients, and—not seeing any nuts listed—gave in and placed the bologna in the cart. I rejoiced! But she scolded me that I'd better make sure to eat all of it since I had been begging her about it. "Yes! Yes!" I said to appease her. Victory was mine! At least for the next six months.

Starting the next day, I arrived in school with my Oscar Mayer bologna and Kraft American cheese sandwich on toasted white Stroehmann bread with the crusts cut off. It sported a little bit of Hellmann's mayo on each side of the bread, two slices of iceberg lettuce, and thinly sliced beefsteak tomatoes. The sandwich had to be cut diagonally across to create two perfect triangular shapes and then carefully placed in a plastic Ziploc sandwich baggie; after that, it went into my Holly Hobbie lunch box. As you can see, I was very particular on how I wanted this experience to come together. Life was grand!

I felt normal having something in my lunchbox that resembled what everyone else had...until one fateful day months later, when that same friend brought something new in her lunchbox that intrigued me. Something called pastrami on rye bread, with a slice of Swiss cheese and some yellow mustard. She even had a damn pickle on the side! My mouth watered just looking at this intriguing combination of flavors. Again, she let me have a bite.

This went on for a week: I took a bite, then two, then three of my friend's sandwiches. This turned into us swapping half of our sandwiches so we could share; eventually, we totally swapped our lunches since she seemed to like mom's bologna and cheese better than she liked her own mom's and I had fallen in love with her pastrami. I didn't have an allergic reaction to the pastrami, so there was no reason to tell my mom what was going on.

But one day, my friend said she no longer wanted my bologna and cheese. "I'm over it!" she declared, and either wanted me to bring in a new sandwich or there would be no more swapping. WTF?!! I had already abandoned my beloved sandwich that I had cried and begged mom to make for me, and now was I supposed to tell her that I had fallen in love with another? Although by that point, I was kinda over eating bologna and cheese.

Terrified to come clean with my mother, I did what any kid in my situation would do: I lied. I ate my snacks and juice at lunchtime, saving the bologna and cheese for later. Then when I got home, I ran upstairs to my room and placed my sandwich carefully behind the radiator in my bedroom, figuring that no one would look there. Voilà! Problem solved!

According to mom's recollections, this must have gone on for at least two weeks, because she noticed a horrible smell all over the house that was driving her crazy. She finally tracked the stinky culprit to my bedroom and then looked behind the radiator. Mortified, she saw a tall stack of my beloved bologna and cheese sandwiches in their plastic bags, which had turned greenish-blue with mold. After that, she gave me the third degree, asking what I had been eating instead. When I confessed, I was scolded for eating food that was *unapproved*.

To teach me my lesson, she took me back to square one and gave me a green chutney sandwich for lunch. "It is healthy, delicious, and has medicinal properties. And it better not be found behind the radiator!" she said. I had never hated my culture so much as when some dumb kid in the lunchroom laughed and said I was eating a mold sandwich.

THE WITCH'S BREWS OF EASTERN MEDICINE

My mom always had a home remedy for everything. Remember the book of witch's brews? Likewise, my Mom used to whip up all kinds of pastes and creams from it, passed down from my grandmother. As a child, for example, she would make me a turmeric and sandalwood paste to apply to my hives to reduce the itch. As much as I complained about the yellow staining of turmeric on my skin, it actually worked.

During the harsh East Coast winters, when the snow was piled high and I'd catch a cold, mom would make her spiced onion brew and repeat "Drink it while it's hot!" at 110 decibels. The brew was made by boiling down onions, ginger, fennel, kadi-patta (curry leaves), cloves, and only God knows what else. It smelled and tasted horrible. But damn, if it wasn't a bona fide cure for the common cold!

Adding turmeric and ginger to hot milk alleviates a cough. Boiling tulsi leaves in water helps a sore throat. And eating fennel or drinking fennel tea helps ease constipation. These sorts of herbal remedies that fight off common colds, upset stomachs, burns, scratches, dry scalp, and more are Ayurvedic remedies and something my parents grew up with in India.

They are made from different plants, herbs, and spices that have medicinal purposes; when mixed together, they make powerful, all-natural treatments for whatever ails you. As a first-generation American child, however, I deemed all of this weird and wanted nothing to do with it as I prioritized my Western culture over my Eastern roots.

In 2008, after being put on 30-plus Western medications, I called my mother and said, "I can't do this anymore." I told her that the drugs were affecting my brain, making me feel lethargic and spacey, as if I couldn't focus on anything. I told mom about a meeting at work where someone had asked me a question and I just sat and stared as if I was completely frozen. "I think it's the side effects from the medicines, mom. They are really strong, and I can't *not* work. What can I do?" That's when we began an open, heart-to-heart conversation about Eastern beliefs on healing.

In her paper titled "Eastern and Western Approaches to Medicine",[59] Julia J. Tsuei, M.D., states that "the development of medicine in Western nations follows the way of hypothetical deduction and the Eastern approach uses the inductive method. The Western approach clearly divides the health from the disease, yet the Eastern approach considers health as a balanced state versus disease as an unbalanced state. The Western approach tends to change the environment and the Eastern way is to prefer to adapt to the environment."

Eastern medicine principles come from many countries, including China, India, and other regions. In China, TCM (or traditional Chinese medicine) is a branch of traditional medicine that is said to be based on more than 3,500 years of Chinese medical practice. TCM uses various forms of herbal medicines, acupuncture techniques, cupping therapy, massage, exercise, and dietary therapy to treat patients.

In India, people have been practicing Ayurveda and homeopathic techniques for centuries. Ayurvedic medicine is one of the world's oldest holistic healing systems—it was developed more than 3,000 years ago in India. It's based on the belief that health and wellness depend on a delicate balance between the mind, body, and spirit. Its main goal is to promote good health, not fight disease, but treatments may be geared toward specific health problems.

As my mother began talking to me about her childhood and the different herbal medicines my grandmother would make when she or her siblings were sick, I started opening my eyes to tradition and began to understand that through these witch's brews, centuries of tradition from our Indian people was being passed down to me. It wasn't that I had to choose *between* East and West—both sides had something beautiful to bring to the table in terms of healing. But unlike the Western side, the Eastern side also focused on healing the mind, spirit, and emotions.

When I told my mother that the harsh prescription medications were making my brain feel like mush, she felt I should consider Ayurvedic and/or homeopathic medicines as a way to treat my allergies. Those techniques would be less harmful overall to my health, she said. "There are many alternative methods out there, the main one being within our own culture. Why don't you open your mind to this now? You have nothing to lose."

She was right—I didn't have anything to lose, as I couldn't stop my Western meds at that immediate moment. Mom telling me to be open was interesting to hear. I felt like I was always the one saying things like that to her!

OPENING MY MIND TO ALTERNATIVE FORMS OF HEALING

Our plan was to find a medical doctor who practiced Ayurvedic and/or homeopathic medicine and give it a try. In parallel, I set out to conduct some research on alternative forms of healing such as naturopathy and integrative medicine just to keep myself informed. We were looking for a whole-body approach, where treatment is focused on the mind and spirit as much as on the body. The ultimate theme and style needed to be bringing the mind, body, and spirit into alignment. If this can be accomplished, then the absence of disease and the presence of optimal health usually follows.

The questions on my mind included:

- What additional options exist to treat my food allergies that are more natural?

- Do any of these options work on getting to the root cause of my food allergies and eradicating them?

- How can I heal my body without causing more harm?

- Is there a way that I can get off the harsh Western meds and completely switch over to something more natural that will manage my allergies?

My mother and I then had conversations with my allergist and my primary care doctor. Both validated that there was no harm in trying other, all-natural ways of managing my food allergies, but they warned me not to go off of my medications at that point as my symptoms might reappear. We agreed. This new path was exciting!

Through my research, I found many other forms of holistic

medicine. While there is much overlap between these disciplines, several important characteristics distinguish these different approaches to healthcare from mainstream approaches.

Naturopathic medicine or naturopathy is a model that crosses a broad spectrum of practices and a wide variety of therapeutic modalities. I learned a great deal by reading an article authored by the True Health Center for Functional Medicine titled "What's the Difference Between Holistic, Naturopathic, Functional and Integrative Medicine?" In it, author Kristine Burke states that "Some naturopaths will adhere to a strict practice of 'nature cure,' focusing only on diet, lifestyle modifications, detoxification and other natural interventions. Other naturopaths will offer additional nonconventional modalities such as acupuncture or homeopathy. At the other end of the spectrum are naturopathic physicians who extensively manipulate the body's physiology and biochemistry by means of botanicals, nutraceuticals, and pharmaceuticals. A majority of naturopathic practitioners incorporate pieces of all these elements in their practice and care for their patients".[60]

Integrative medicine is a model of healthcare in which conventional medicine is integrated with nonconventional or alternative modalities (such as herbs, homeopathy, chiropractic, acupuncture, etc.). This is an area I knew a little about as I had already tried some of these methods before. Dr. Andrew Weil states that "Integrative medicine is a healing-oriented medicine that takes account of the whole person (body, mind, and spirit), including all aspects of lifestyle. It emphasizes the therapeutic relationship and makes use of all appropriate therapies, both conventional and alternative".[61] This seemed to resonate the most with me in terms of a methodology.

Ayurvedic medicine is based on the notion that good health depends on the balance between mind, body, and spirit. It focuses on restoring balance in the body through a personalized plan that can include massage, specialized diets, herbs, aromatherapy, and exercise. According to Ayurvedic theory, everyone is made up of a combination of five elements: air, water, fire, earth, and space. These elements combine in the body to form three energies or life forces called doshas: Vata, Kapha, and Pitta. Although each person has a unique mix of the three doshas, one dosha is usually the most influential. Each type of dosha has a unique set of characteristics, and a person's body type depends on their dosha's physical and emotional attributes. To maintain good health and state of mind, it is necessary to know your dosha so that you can pursue a suitable diet, exercise, and lifestyle pattern.

In Ayurveda, the balance of a person's doshas is thought to explain some of his or her individual differences and the likelihood of illness. An imbalanced dosha is believed to interrupt the natural flow of vital energy, or prana. This disrupted energy flow is thought to impair digestion and allow the buildup of body waste or ama, which further impairs energy and digestion. In my specific situation, if there was a lot of fire inside of me in the form of toxins, it could manifest as hives all over my body. The hives were the manifestation of the toxins trying to flush out of my system.

All of this information gave me hope that I would not have to rely solely on Western meds to manage my allergies. Considering that I was trying to clean up my life in both the literal and figurative sense, all-natural herbal remedies, supplements, and practices seemed like a great fit to complement my current protocol. I hoped they would one day become my *main* protocol.

AYURVEDIC MEDICINE AS A NEW PATH

Through our Big Fat Indian Network, mom received a referral to a medical doctor who also practiced Ayurveda. (We set up a virtual initial consult as the doctor was in Maryland.) She asked me very detailed questions about my health, diet, lifestyle, and sex life and had already reviewed my health history and data from recent tests. We conversed about the principles of Ayurveda and setting my expectations about the practice. In Ayurveda, there is a term called "satmya" that means tolerance; "asatmy" means intolerance. This tolerance or intolerance can be toward any medicine, food, weather, or even any habits. Ayurveda believes that asatmya is a result of weak or imbalanced agni (digestive fire). A weak agni means there is ama (toxin) formation in the body. Therefore, as a principle, allergies are more common in people with ama in their system.

With new testing, my Ayurvedic doctor's conclusion was that my predominant dosha was Pitta, or fire. The aggravating causes of a Pitta-related allergy are foods that are spicy, sour, and/or salty. Factors such as extreme hot weather can also be triggers. Symptoms include red rash, dermatitis, eczema, redness of the skin, heartburn, acidity, nausea, burning, etc. The Pitta dosha's most important organs are the skin, eyes, digestive system, liver, and spleen. This information felt on point when we discussed my history and the hive situations I had had.

Like Western medicine, Ayurveda believes in avoiding all allergens in everyday life and also during detoxification. So, the plan we agreed to was the following:

· Avoid foods causing Pitta allergic reactions.

- Reduce sweet, sour, and salty foods in favor of foods that were pungent (i.e., spicy foods like chilies, radishes, raw garlic), astringent (i.e., legumes, vegetables, apples), and bitter.

- Stay out of extreme heat conditions. (Boo! I love the beach...)

- Take Ayurvedic herbs to treat Pitta-related allergies.

- Drink herbal teas with ingredients such as fennel, turmeric, ginger, and saffron and juices such as coriander juice and fresh coconut water.

- Utilize sandalwood and neem on my hives, which are all-natural ingredients that can reduce the redness and itch.

- Replace all butter, margarine, and vegetable oil in my house with better alternatives, including ghee. The good news was that I was already doing this!

The doctor also prescribed taking Ayurvedic herbs that promoted the healthy elimination of natural toxins. These herbs offered antioxidant properties, balanced the female hormones, had soothing effects on the digestive tract and the healthy peristalsis of the bowels, and gave moisturizing support of the respiratory tract. Additionally, they provided many other benefits for the immune system, liver, kidneys, and skin.

The herbs I took were shatavari, guduchi, triphala, brahmi, neem, and manjistha. During my first year of treatment, the doctor played around with the dosages of these herbs (which came in pill and loose-leaf formats) to find the right combination.

In addition to this, I found a local salon that specialized in Eastern forms of massage therapy. I began the arduous task of getting a monthly massage to aid in overall circulation and removal of toxins. It was a very hard job to lie on a massage table and have someone pamper you—but if someone has to do it, it may as well be me! For several months, I went for an Abhyanga massage with a Shirodhara treatment every week. Abhyanga is a massage of the body with dosha-specific, warmed, herb-infused oil. The oil typically is premixed with herbs for specific conditions. In the case of my Pitta dosha, Ayurvedic medicine would use coconut and sunflower oil. The spa I went to let me purchase the oil so that I could do a massage at home three to four times a week to restore the balance of my doshas and enhance my well-being and longevity. We were trying to calm my Pitta dosha and bring balance to all three. With the massage, I benefited from improving my circulation, moving my lymphatic system, aiding the detoxification process, and stimulating my internal organs.

Shirodara is an Ayurvedic therapy that balances and stabilizes the mind. During this treatment, I would lie down on a massage table with my eyes covered while a specially prepared warm herbal oil was poured in a thin, steady stream directly onto my forehead onto the third-eye chakra, known as being the center of intuition and foresight. This focal point is a key juncture for nerves and tissues and also the circulation of vital life force. The oil would then stream backwards down into my hair and the masseuse would give me a head massage. Like I said, rough times...

We had a plan for incorporating Ayurvedic medicine into my daily life, and we worked this plan in parallel with my Western medications. All of this was actually very exciting and—finally!—relaxing. This hybrid process allowed me to see the beautiful touchpoints of Eastern medicine and health and why my mother had always used her home remedies on us.

CONNECTING THE DOTS IN ALTERNATIVE MEDICINES

During the decade following my 2008 incident, I utilized both Ayurvedic and functional medicine in parallel since they both seek to identify the underlying cause of disease rather than prescribe a cure for the symptom alone. They both maintain balance in the body and mind, and they both foster a sense of well-being through being attuned to one's nutrition, habitual patterns of eating and drinking, lifestyle, exercise, sleep, hygiene, and stress management practices. They also look at the human body as a complete system and view symptoms as being offshoots of deeper, systemic issues.

Ayurveda is particularly attuned to the quality and quantity of foods consumed, including what time you eat and your habitual patterns of eating and eliminating. It is also focused on our core beliefs about ourselves and our sense of meaning in the world. Lastly, Ayurveda is focused on the basic metabolic mechanisms that drive our energy levels. Holistically, all of this spoke to me.

It's important to note that when I set out to explore Ayurveda and functional medicine, I was still on Western meds, and I wasn't sure whether I was ever going to be able to completely get off of those meds and manage my food allergies and health more naturally.

BEGINNING TO SEE NEW RESULTS

By the end of 2010, just two years after my emergent incident, I was able to completely get off Western medications. Woo-hoo! I began making the transition to Ayurvedic herbs during my year of hives and stayed on them for several years. Then, once I began working with a functional medicine doctor, I swapped out some of the Ayurvedic herbs for others. This was a personalized plan for me, working with multiple medical professionals who were invested in me, and a part of my support team.

I was overjoyed to get off the last Western medication I had been taking to treat my food allergies! If I did get sick and required some form of Western medication, I didn't say no, although I would first ask if there was something all-natural I could use instead. Sometimes there was sometimes there wasn't. Being open to things also comes with compromise.

Today, I continue to use all-natural herbal supplements as prescribed by my Ayurvedic doctor and my functional medicine doctor to manage my holistic health. I have seen many improvements in my skin, weight, and overall health by incorporating these into my daily life, the biggest one being that I am finally working proactively to prevent ailments and help ease symptoms of my chronic disease. This has allowed for much greater inner peace than I had ever experienced before.

HOW YOU CAN EXPAND YOUR AWARENESS TO HEALING

Your health is unique and deserves a personalized focus, a philosophy that gets to the root of your problem and doesn't just suppress your symptoms. Everyone who has food allergies wants to be rid of them! It's not like we love eliminating a gazillion foods or being scared of eating or that we want to take harsh meds for the rest of our lives.

BEING SAFE IS ABOUT HAVING MULTIPLE OPTIONS AT YOUR FINGERTIPS AT ALL TIMES AND NOT RELYING ON ONE METHOD ONLY.

Being safe is also about utilizing natural products that can help you heal, and not staying on genetically modified and/or pharmaceutical-grade products for your entire life.

To begin expanding your awareness to other forms of healing, try the following:

Step One: Look Deep Within. Ask yourself the following questions and write them down in your journal. Once you begin this process, you will start to ideate more questions on your own.

- How would you prioritize transforming your health on a scale of 1, 2, or 3, with 1 being the highest priority? Why did you assign it this priority?

- What is your level of dedication to transforming your health and well-being? Think of this on a scale of "I'll get to it when I can" to "I am dedicated to achieving optimal health in everything I do in my life."

- Is it important that you only put items into or onto your body that do not harm it in other ways? Why?

- What is holding you back from entertaining other, more holistic ways of managing your health?

- How can you begin to utilize natural products in your food, lifestyle, and environment, everyday? What are those products? Create a list of items that you current eat/use and write down alternative options for each.

- Do you take vitamins and/or herbal supplements that assist in managing your food allergies? If you don't, start asking your doctor about this.

Step Two: Find the Right Medical Professional. Given my severe allergy situation, it was important to me that when I found the right Ayurvedic or functional medicine doctor, they also were an M.D. This was my personal preference, although I am positive that many other holistic professionals who are licensed and certified but who are not M.D.s can likewise make a positive impact in your life. Begin with your own allergist and primary care doctors and find out if they have someone on their staff who treats allergies more holistically or if they can refer you to someone who does. In the process of finding the holistic health professional to work with, you'll learn so much about your body! Not to mention the medical philosophies, types of tests, and data that you will begin to gain knowledge about from working with a holistic practitioner.

Step Three: Edit Your World...Slowly. As with all things, don't rush into alternative forms of healing your food allergies. Take this process at your own pace and absolutely do not put a time limit on it. Instead, think of it as something you're doing to achieve your North Star. If you are on a medical protocol to manage your food allergies, ask your holistic practitioners to explore the proper supplements that will benefit you. Ask what supplements you can utilize to heal your gut. This process is a very personalized regimen for your body, so the microsteps that you take in the areas of food, lifestyle, and environment should not add stress to your life! On the contrary, hopefully they will add joy that you are taking care of your health in a cleaner way.

We live in an amazing world where much new science has emerged over the past decade or so related to managing and ridding oneself of food allergies. We are learning more about the power of plants to heal ailments like food allergies; we hear stories of people who made drastic changes in just their diet and exercise and were able to rid themselves of cancers. Expanding your mind to new forms of healing your food allergies can be an adventure of growth. Take some time to consider joining the ranks of those healing themselves holistically.

If you are on a journey of learning and growth as I was when I was creating the *Three to Be™ Program*, begin by speaking with your allergist about undertaking other, more natural forms of healing food allergies in addition to what you are doing already. Have a discussion about functional medicine, Ayurveda, or even integrative medicine. Involve them in this process as I did. Every time I tried a new herb, I let my allergist and primary care doctor know ahead of time to get their thoughts. Opening yourself up to other forms of healing also means having an open discussion with your medical support team about why you are interested in this to begin with. Be proactive. Don't wait for someone to prescribe the next medication after an incident! Get ahead of the game in order to hit your North Star.

THE NET NET

Learning about different cultures helps us break down barriers and overcome stereotypes. It influences our views, values, and hopes and is a way to be empathetic to others as you forge relationships in the process.

For most of my young life, I pooh-poohed my own Indian culture and the traditions it brought because I wanted to fit into the American world I was born into. Through health hardships, I realized this was just plain silly and that the two sides of my life didn't need to compete. Instead, I could take the greatest parts of both and combine them to create a unique perspective that opened me up to new ways of living.

REMEMBER, THERE IS NO ONE WAY TO DO YOU. YOU ARE MADE UP OF MULTIPLE UNIQUE QUALITIES, AND YOUR TREATMENT OPTIONS SHOULD BE, TOO.

Work with different doctors who have a diverse yet integrating philosophies to determine what is going on. From there, it's up to you on how you want to proceed.

For me, I was drowning in Western medications all of my life that made me feel shitty all-around. When I proclaimed, "No more!" back in 2008, I meant no more visits to the hospital and no more me putting crap into my body that could harm me in other ways. I found that exploring different cultural practices for health and healing opened my mind's eye to the possibility that I could one day defeat the odds and hit my North Star of getting rid of my food allergies.

The process involved an exploration of my culture, generations of traditions, and science mapped onto nontraditional methods. A *healthy* human being is incredibly complex. Add on an illness or imbalance, and that complexity grows exponentially. I was not striving for perfect health in this process because I don't believe it exists. We are works in progress in life and in health. This process was about balance. All of the various medical approaches have their merits, but the obvious choice for me was an approach that encompassed all of them while simultaneously using systems biology to unravel our complex networks and seek out the root cause of the illness. Given that I had *not* been doing this at all before, it was a big change for me.

An EpiPen® and a rescue inhaler are still in my purse at all times in case of dire emergencies. But my mind is at peace knowing that I'm not pumping strong medications into my body daily, that are masking symptoms and causing long-term effects. My body and mind are healthier because I know where each ingredient I consume came from. My spirit and emotions are alive again because I know that I am taking daily microsteps to reach my North Star and eradicate my issues.

So, where do we go from here? Along with my exploration of Ayurvedic medicine, I began learning about the relationship of food to health and Ayurvedic cooking. Cooking is the number one thing you can do to be healthy and be safe living with food allergies. In "Chapter 9: Cooking Consciously," I wrap up our journey of being safe by talking about the relationships we have with foods and their sources, and why that is so important when living with food allergies. Cooking is everything from pulling together a sandwich to creating an entire meal from scratch. Doing this with intention is what our next chapter is all about. Yum, yum!

Stories of Wisdom on Cooking Consciously

What does conscious food entrepreneurship mean to you and what led you to this path?

Colleen Kavanaugh, CEO and Founder of Zego Foods

"Like many parents, I struggled to balance my kids' dietary restrictions and their school's ban on nuts with my desire for delicious, nourishing, and convenient foods. The allergy-safe options I found in stores didn't back their claims with testing and were full of processed ingredients. I wanted safe foods that supported my kids' short- and long-term health.

So, I started my company, ZEGO, to make nutritious, delicious products that meet the needs of most special diets. We test for allergen and gluten cross-contact regularly and link the test results to each package. I learned many ingredients have hidden toxins also, like pesticides and heavy metals that damage your health. So we set quality standards and expanded our purity testing and transparency to those as well.

We are leading the way to set a new standard across the food industry: consumers have a right to know if there are hidden toxins in their food. This transparency will force the industry to clean up the food supply chain, from farming to processing to packaging.

Having a mission greater than your product is critical, but it's just one part of conscious food entrepreneurship. I think beyond filling a gap in the marketplace. My goal is continuous improvement in all aspects of the company, from source to the shelf to the employee manual. I feel conscious food entrepreneurship should be the only option for emerging food companies. And, everyone has to be part of the solution, including investors. We can build responsible brands, but conscious capital has to be available to support them."

NINE

Cooking Consciously

"... food is about more than cooking; it's about geography, history, agriculture, tradition, art, anthropology — and nature, of course..."

— ALICE WATERS

LEARNINGS

In this chapter, we'll explore how your relationship with food is connected to mindset, and how it can change from being negative to being healthy and mindful. You'll learn:

- Holistic health is focused on cooking and eating for health above all else.

- Redefining and redesigning your relationship with food can save your life.

- The conscious decisions you make around food will allow your health *and* our planet's health to thrive.

MY EARLY YEARS

In India, people either go to the market daily or the market comes to you. It's a mix of people scurrying around, pointing at things and bartering, while live animals are slaughtered right in front of you. This was all very exciting to me as a young child visiting relatives because I saw none of this at the local Acme Market—there, everything was quiet, pristine, and prepackaged in Styrofoam.

During a trip to India in my youth, I was sitting in my grandparent's living room when I heard a woman outside yelling at the top of her lungs, saying something I couldn't understand. I jumped up and ran to the balcony, put down the footstool, and stood on it to see what the commotion was. I saw a woman walking down the street with a huge basket on top of her head. The woman was super skinny, old, and so wrinkly that she looked like she had been lying on the beach for ten hours too long.

I watched in awe as my grandmother walked up next to me, yelled something down to this lady, and motioned her to come upstairs. I screamed in excitement! Who was this stranger who was going to carry that basket up all five flights of stairs to the top floor where my grandparents lived?

I waited beside my grandmother when she opened the door and saw her: the Bhaji Walee. That actually wasn't her name, though. Translated, it means "the vegetable lady," and it describes what she was carrying in the basket on her head. My grandmother shooed me out of the way and invited the Bhaji Walee into our kitchen, pouring her a cup of chai and beginning a conversation about purchasing vegetables. My heart was beating so fast I thought it was going to pop out of my chest.

Once in the kitchen, the woman removed the basket from her head and placed it on the floor to reveal an array of fresh vegetables—eggplant, cauliflower, okra—and a small scale. These vegetables came from farms in India, and this lady's job was to walk through neighborhoods and sell out her basket before repeating the same thing the next day.

I began pointing to vegetables that I wanted to eat. We proceeded to order as the woman weighed each one on her scale and stated its price. And then the dance began. Like a scene out of *Wall Street* (one of the greatest movies of all time) starring Michael Douglas, where traders on the floor of the New York Stock Exchange are shouting out God knows what, I witnessed hands in the air and raised voices. I tried to decipher the numbers, prices, and calculations, hearing "No no!" from my grandmother followed by another haggle of compromise from the Bhaji Walee.

Finally, an agreement was made. The lady wrapped up the basket, put it back on her head, and elegantly swooshed out of the door and down the stairs as I ran back to the balcony window and hopped up on the footstool to see where she was going next. She continued yelling and walking down the street, looking for her next sale. But then for a second, she paused and looked up at me.

I waved; she smiled. I had just witnessed pure magic.

Similar to the Bhaji Walee, there was a Dana Walee and a Masa Walee, or "grain lady" and "fish lady" respectively. The Masa Walee came to Grandma's house with the fresh catch of the day and would even scale the fish for us before she left. I would rant on for hours about all of this to the rest of my family when they came home. I'd explain how after the Walees had left, my grandmother and I would walk around the corner to buy spices and then I helped her make dinner for the night. No one seemed overly interested in my stories, but I didn't care! This scenario never happened in America, and it was my first introduction to the term "farm to fork."

However, despite my foodie upbringing, by the time 2008 rolled around, I was eating out more than I was cooking at home. Not because I wanted to, but because I was traveling 50 percent of the time for work, and wineing and dining clients. When I was at home, it felt difficult to keep up with menu planning and making the traditional dishes I loved so much in the small amount of time left to myself. It was way easier to order a deelish curry from the local Indian restaurant! My diet at the time wasn't necessarily nutritious per se—I was eating more protein than vegetables for sure and I loved me some carbs! Of course, I was still reading labels for allergic ingredients, but in retrospect, I cannot say I was eating very healthily. Rather, I was just getting by.

I had a bad habit of undereating and not getting enough calories which wasn't great for my metabolism; sometimes I even drank my calories with a protein shake and then had late-night pizza with friends. Such was the life of a bachelorette. When I did cook, I shopped at markets like Trader Joe's and Whole Foods, often buying prepackaged food that just needed some spicing or dressing up for flavor. On weekends when I had more time, I would prepare a home-cooked meal and invite friends over to share. We would indulge in many rich foods and drinks as a treat after a long work week.

There was no balance and not much thought put into my cooking in 2008 aside from making sure there were no nuts or other allergic items in my food. I can't say that I had full knowledge of what else was in what I was eating. Meaning, I wasn't looking at the nutritional facts label (or any other label) much, so I didn't know if my food was healthy or what the sources of the ingredients were. My life at the time was fast, fast, fast! As if I were on autopilot, I had a bad habit of pulling together meals and eating them quickly with no other thought.

But when I left the emergency room in 2008, I vowed to slow down and say goodbye to my old ways. I set out to relearn everything related to cooking.

LEARNING HOW TO COOK, AGAIN

Now that you've gotten to know me, you've probably guessed that I sat down and had a strategy session with myself about the state of my cooking. The first concept I wrote on the whiteboard was, "What is my current relationship with food and how does that need to change?" Changing was a necessity, not an option; learning how to cook properly wasn't a desire, it was a dire need. With copious amounts of thinking and journaling, I realized that my relationship with food at the time was about *living to eat*. I wanted to get to the reverse of that: *eating to live*. Which meant looking at my cooking processes and choices through a different lens without giving up my foodie status.

Of course I ate healthy food, but mainly because I didn't want to become fat. I had equated food with abundance—and with the wrong definition of the word. For example, when I went for a long run, I would often reward myself with a huge bowl of spaghetti afterward. The pasta was boxed, and the sauce was from a jar. In other words, they were processed foods. Or sometimes I snarfed down a burger, fries (not made in peanut oil), and a shake. These foods satisfied my brain more than my tummy—I viewed them as something I deserved because I had just completed a ten-mile run. I remember joking with friends that I worked out so that I could eat whatever I wanted. The statement wasn't really that off. *Living to eat* was an unhealthy loop, and my food choices at the time included lots of low-quality, overly rich foods that weren't good for me. My head was not on straight about all of this as it related to my allergies and overall health, and that needed to change.

Eating to live was a bigger concept than just food—it was about the components of what I ate being nutritious and healing for me *and* the planet. As I was looking at my health holistically, I needed to look at my relationship with food in the same way. I wrote "holistic health = holistic nutrition" on my whiteboard. This statement meant me having an understanding of a few things:

- What was holistic nutrition and how did it apply to my food allergy situation?

- Which specific foods were nourishing to my overall health today and for the future?

- What were the sources of those foods?

- What were the conscious decisions I needed to make to support all of the above?

By understanding this information, I could begin to build a new and different relationship with food that simultaneously satisfied and healed me. And I could think about abundance in terms of being grateful for the bounty of foods that I *could* eat.

EMPHASIZING HOLISTIC NUTRITION

Holistic nutrition requires a whole-life approach: when and where you eat, where your food comes from, and incorporates not only the body but also the mind and spirit as well. The National Association of Nutrition Professionals states, "The philosophy of holistic nutrition is that one's health is an expression of the complex interplay between the physical and chemical, mental and emotional, as well as spiritual and environmental aspects of one's life and being".[62] So, holistic nutrition is about eating healthy food that's as close to its natural state as possible in order to achieve optimum health and well-being. It's an approach to eating that very consciously considers *everything* we eat and focuses on eating for our health above all else.

This was a great path to take with respect to my food allergies, because the hallmarks of holistic nutrition include eating unrefined, unprocessed, organic, and locally grown whole foods. By definition, that was where my focus needed to be when I was purchasing food in markets and cooking it at home.

With a changed mindset, I made a few conscious decisions going forward:

Step One: No Outside Food. I completely stopped eating out for one year. I needed to heal my body and reset, and to do that, I had to know exactly every single ingredient that was going into my body and where it came from. There were no exceptions here, not even on my birthday.

Step Two: Prioritize Certain Food Labels. I decided to only eat food with labels that said "unrefined," "unprocessed," "USDA organic," "locally grown," "Non-GMO Project Verified," "American grass-fed," or "sustainable." I was also interested in Fair Trade, non-MSG, and gluten-free foods. Why did I make this decision? Because I wanted to stop the madness of consciously adding toxins to my body by eating things that were not good for me or the planet.

In working with my functional medicine doctor and my Ayurvedic doctor and in partnership with a nutritionist, I created a spreadsheet of brands and foods whose ingredients would fit into my plan of holistic nutrition. My spreadsheet made me feel like a mad scientist, and I loved it! We are so blessed to have companies working on creating food that doesn't make us sick and that give us alternatives to falling prey to the growing number of food-related diseases in America. Companies like Enjoy Life Foods®, Beyond Meat Foods, Banza, ZEGO, and purely elizabeth are driven by purpose, holistic health, and nutrition. They provide delicious options and especially for people with severe food allergies. I could not be more grateful to all of the people at each of these companies who tirelessly work on helping others to be healthy and safe.

TRYING AN AYURVEDIC DIET

The American College of Healthcare Sciences states that "Holistic nutrition can also include a specific cultural philosophy—like Ayurveda or Traditional Chinese Medicine—or a specific diet—such as ancestral foods, raw foods, cleansing, vegetarianism, or anti-inflammatory".[63]

Ayurveda believes that all diseases come from the stomach and that our health depends not only on what type of food we eat, but also on the ability of our body to digest and absorb these foods. The pillars of Ayurvedic nutrition are food, exercise, sleep, and emotional wellness, all necessary components for keeping energy balanced and achieving good health. Ayurveda recommends having a spiritual relationship with food, because what you put into your vessel (you) is the fuel and energy you need to prosper in life, achieve your goals, and live a healthy and fit life.

In an Ayurvedic diet, all six tastes need to be present for a balanced meal. They are: sweet, salty, sour, pungent, bitter, and astringent (acidic). So, depending on your dosha, you need to incorporate a certain amount of each on your plate. It's all about having balance in order to promote proper digestion and keep your energy from being aggravated. The timing of when you eat each meal is also very important in an Ayurvedic diet, plus you're not supposed to eat three hours before sleeping. (Something I was famous for!)

Step Three: Eat According to My Dosha. I made a conscious decision to incorporate the following whole foods into my diet that were specific to my Pitta dosha. I specifically sought out the organic versions of all items and thank God I wasn't allergic to any form of them!

- **Fruit:** sweet apples, berries, grapes, pears, plums, pomegranates, watermelon.

- **Vegetables:** artichoke, asparagus, broccoli, cabbage, cauliflower, kale, leafy greens, lettuce, mushrooms, peas, peppers, spaghetti squash, zucchini.

- **Grains:** amaranth, couscous, oat bran, quinoa, wild rice.

- **Legumes:** chickpeas, lentils (red and brown), peas, pinto beans, white beans.

- **Dairy:** ghee, cottage cheese, goat cheese.

- **Protein:** freshwater fish, tempeh, tofu.

- **Nuts and seeds:** coconut, flaxseeds, sunflower seeds.

The items on this list changed based on seasonality, the results of my food allergy testing, and yearly checkups with my Ayurvedic doctor to diagnose the strength of my agni and the degree of my dosha predominance. These items went into my spreadsheet as ingredients that I would primarily cook with. It was actually a fun process to try to figure out how to incorporate these into some of my favorite dishes! My cooking was taking on a whole new life, one that felt clean and healthy and like it was healing me for the first time in my life.

GIVING PLANT-BASED A CHANCE

Ironically, my parents had grown up on a plant-based diet—their meals in India were mainly vegetables and grains mixed with herbs and spices. Fish and meat were something you only ate on special occasions. My mom always made a lot of delicious Indian vegetarian dishes when I was a kid, but we were carnivores, which came more from our American culture. As a child, I didn't think about where that meat came from or what effect it was having on my body or the planet.

These were not subjects discussed in health class, either! But after 2008, I began thinking hard about this subject just as mainstream media was starting to talk about climate change and the role of our food in our planet's health.

"Food is the single strongest lever to optimize human health and environmental sustainability on Earth",[64] according to the EAT Lancet Commission report. "Food systems have environmental impacts along the entire supply chain from production to processing and retail, and furthermore reach beyond human and environmental health by also affecting society, culture, economy, and animal health and welfare." This report goes deep into the direct correlation between our diet choices and planetary health and the corresponding conscious decisions we must make. Because "Without action... today's children will inherit a planet that has been severely degraded and where much of the population will increasingly suffer from malnutrition and preventable disease."

> *AS SOMEONE WHO IS DRIVEN BY LEGACY AND LEAVING THE PLANET A BETTER PLACE FOR FUTURE GENERATIONS, IT REALLY HIT ME HARD TO THINK ABOUT THE POSITIVE IMPACT I COULD MAKE ON MY OWN HEALTH AND FOR THE PLANET JUST BY MAKING SOME DIETARY SHIFTS.*

But going plant-based scared the bejeezus out of me! Just cutting out red meat was already a big step. Going a full 180 degrees was even scarier, but I had hope.

Katherine D. McManus, M.S., R.D., L.D.N. and contributor to Harvard Health Publishing at Harvard Medical School, states, "Plant-based or plant-forward eating patterns focus on foods primarily from plants. This includes not only fruits and vegetables, but also nuts, seeds, oils, whole grains, legumes, and beans. It doesn't mean that you are vegetarian or vegan and never eat meat or dairy. Rather, you are proportionately choosing more of your foods from plant sources".[65]

This made sense on so many levels! And it was easy to digest, if you will. Today, there are a plethora of plant-based food options, like alternatives for meat, milk, pasta, ice cream, yogurt, and even bacon! As a foodie, tasting is believing. If it doesn't taste exactly the same or very close to it, I'm out. When I first tried Daiya cheese in 2008, I felt it was horrible. But trying it again ten years later, wowza! Those R&D people were really hard at work, because today it tastes exactly like real cheese, plus its usage is just about at a 1:1 ratio, where it melts and cooks the same way real cheese does. Why would I even bother buying real cheese if I could cook with a product that had amazing flavor and form and was better for my health and the planet's health? Thanks, Daiya.

Step Four: Go Plant-Based. I made another conscious decision to slowly change my diet to plant-based, and I placed a priority on purchasing plant-based ingredients and foods to the extent that I could given my allergies. Having been a carnivore my entire life, this didn't happen overnight. But I embraced it and began with not buying red meat; then I ate meat less often; then I didn't eat meat at all for many months. Because many plant-based foods are made with tree nuts and legumes, I kept readjusting and finding alternative options once again.

The plant-based movement is something that every person on this planet needs to pay attention to. Doing my own research to understand the science behind how climate change is affected by the daily choices we make (right down to the level of our food choices!) was incredibly eye-opening and humbling. For so long, I had thought that having severe food allergies would make me *not* a good candidate for pursuing a plant-based diet, and that may have been true at some point. But today, there is nothing stopping any of us from leaving this planet healthy and thriving for future generations!

HOW YOU CAN BEGIN TO COOK CONSCIOUSLY

Cooking is what you make of it, and it does not have to be intimidating. If you make the best damn bologna and cheese sandwich with all the fixings—well, then that's cooking, and don't let anyone tell you it's not! Whether you chopped the onion or bought a pre-cut onion and then mixed it with other ingredients—it's all cooking! Cooking takes thought, practice, and lots of love—the latter *is* the essence of cooking. Learning to cook will literally save your life, because then you will begin to have in-depth knowledge about every ingredient that goes into your body. Cooking consciously will transform your life, because a personalized food plan that includes clean, alternative products eaten at the right times will help solidify proper gut health while providing many other health benefits that also benefit the environment.

Step One: Dig into the Bowl of your Soul. I love starting off with theory—in this case, cooking theory. Ask yourself the following questions and write your answers in your journal.

- What is your relationship with food? Do you live to eat or eat to live?

- What does cooking consciously mean to you?

- Write a list of the top 5 ways you can begin to cook consciously.

- How dedicated are you to learning on a scale of 1, 2, or 3, with 1 being the highest priority? Why did you assign it this priority?

- How has eating out impacted your health?

- Which labels are important for your food allergies and for healthy, conscious eating? Categorize them into "approved" and "avoid" categories.

- What dish(es) do you crave and would love to find an allergy-free option for, one that would be healthier for you and the planet? Start a list and begin finding recipes online and in cookbooks. Then determine which allergy and planet friendly ingredients you can utilize to bring it to life!

Step Two: Expand your Beliefs, Patterns, and Habits. Begin by asking yourself, "What microsteps can I take to change my eating that will greatly benefit my overall health?" Do away with the belief that certain foods just won't taste the same or good—that is just not the case. Discovering that shirataki noodles are low in carbs and calories and are free of nuts, gluten, wheat, dairy, and tofu is a huge benefit for your food allergies, and they taste great! Pasta made from cauliflower, rice flour, or pea proteins (boxed or fresh) are equally as pliable and delicious.

By trying new, more natural ingredients and different methods of cooking, you are already expanding your old beliefs, patterns, and habits. Make sure to make these conscious decisions and work every day to stick with them. They can be as small as "I will no longer eat at fast-food joints" to as big as "I'm completely switching to plant-based as of today." When you think about food and nutrition holistically, you'll know that taking small, daily steps to actually make these changes will keep you safe and healthy. And the moment you begin to consciously shift your choices, you'll see changes in your skin and your digestion and how you feel overall.

Step Three: Balance Cooking at Home and Eating Out. Eating out at a restaurant with family and friends is one of life's greatest joys and should always be a (balanced) possibility for someone managing food allergies, but you'll need to determine what mix works best for you. For example, after my 2008 incident, I consciously chose not to eat out at any restaurant for over one year until I had healed from my allergies. It was not as hard as you would think—it just required a lot of planning and dinner parties at home. When eating out, in addition to avoiding items you're allergic to, try to make the conscious choice of choosing restaurants that also consciously cook. The only way to know this is to contact the restaurant and ask how they design their menus, or you can follow the chef on social media and learn more about their philosophies and cooking practices.

THE NET NET

Cooking is life! It is a way for humans to connect with love and as a community. Learning how to cook kept me safe in situations where I didn't have other options, because then I was able to pull something together for myself. It also gave me the ability to learn and carry forward my family traditions. The National Institute of Health states that "...cooking skills are increasingly included in strategies to prevent and reduce chronic diet-related diseases and obesity".[66] I can tell you from firsthand experience that it never matters when you start, only that you do.

Understanding the essence of food, what its purpose is for your body, and what works or doesn't work for you is essential to living with food allergies. Making conscious decisions about what food you put into your body and where it comes from is also essential to living with food allergies. It's equally as essential for our planetary health.

In the COVID-19 world, the popularity of fast food delivery from Uber Eats and DoorDash skyrocketed. Most diets went berserk, people ordered in many meals, and waistlines and health went to shit in an already shitty year. As I have learned from many friends, stress eating is a real thing and a big issue for many, especially when they're isolated in their house for months at a time. But it doesn't have to be that way! When you are pushed up against the wall is exactly when you need to slow down, think, and make conscious decisions about what foods you want to put into your body. Enjoying a diet of fresh, properly sourced foods that you cook yourself is the best way to keep your body healthy and safe from harm. Changing to a more holistic way of eating (such as an Ayurvedic diet) will allow you to actually heal from the inside out, with foods that taste amazing and expand your mind.

So, where do we go from here? Now you have three additional tools in your pocket to keep yourself safe by using a holistic health perspective. You began by creating a safe-care plan, then you used your changed mindset to explore additional ways of healing your body that are more natural and better for the long-run, and now you're learning how to cook by making conscious decisions. Look at you!

Up to this point, the primary focus of the *Three to Be™ Program* has been inward—you've been defining or redefining how to be healthy and be safe. As we move into the fourth and final area of this book, I will show you how I took everything I learned and began to share it with the world. It was time to set myself free from years of trauma, hostility, and everything else terrible about living life with food allergies and begin to let go. This was my time to be a beacon of hope for others and begin to thrive myself.

To me, freedom meant being fearless with consciousness. It was freeing to take that first step in this entire program even though I didn't know where I was going to end up. With my North Star guiding me, I was conducting my life in a different way—one that was finally serving me—and I was healing. The final part of this book, "Part IV: Be Well," describes my journey toward beginning to thrive by helping others.

PART IV

Be Well

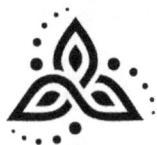

THREE TO BE

Healthy	Safe	Well
Step 1 CHANGING MINDSET	**Step 4** CREATING A SAFE-CARE PLAN	**Step 7** **LEARNING TO ADVOCATE**
Step 2 FINDING A NORTH STAR	**Step 5** EXPANDING AWARENESS TO HEALING	**Step 8** **DESIGNING A FOOD ALLERGY CARD**
Step 3 BUILDING A SUPPORT TEAM	**Step 6** COOKING CONSCIOUSLY	**Step 9** **HUMANIZING FOOD ALLERGIES**

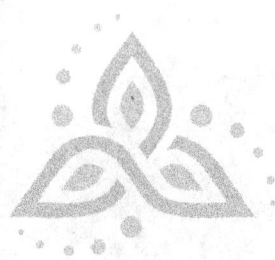

Being well is the ultimate experience of health, happiness, and prosperity that my parents wished for their children.

> **THROUGH THIS TRANSFORMATIONAL PROCESS, I DEFINED "BEING WELL" AS MY BODY, MIND, SPIRIT, AND EMOTIONS IN ALIGNMENT AND PRODUCING A HARMONIOUS FEELING OF WELL-BEING THAT ALLOWS ME TO THRIVE.**

I created this statement to remind myself why the hell I was doing all of this to begin with! Finally, I was on the right path with a life theme I believed in. In these final three steps of the *Three to Be™ Program,* we'll apply everything we've learned forward to hit our North Stars.

Being well is about becoming empowered, but it's also about empowering others around you. In one of the greatest scenes of all time from the Oscar-winning movie *Jerry Maguire,* Tom Cruise as Jerry passionately states to his footballer client, Rod Tidwell, "Help me help *you.*" What Jerry was trying to get across to Rod was that through openness, communication, and working together, both people could thrive.

Isn't that what we're all here for? To help and love one another? Jerry wanted to get into Rod's soul and understand him in order to help him, because even though Rod acted like an ass at times, Jerry still cared about him. This resonated with having food allergies, because unless I were to live in a bubble, I had to interact with other humans in some capacity (possibly every day), and I didn't want those interactions to be negative. If I wanted good will to come to me, I first had to put it out into the world and help others.

Being well was also about putting my vulnerability to the test by not being afraid to advocate for myself or start a dialogue with someone new around my health and well-being. In order to fulfill the three steps I needed to be well, I thought about what tools would "Help me help *you*," as Jerry had said. How could I take all of the knowledge I had acquired thus far and offer it to the world? Eventually, after much thought, I came up with the notion of humanizing food allergies.

Humanizing is about making things easier for humans to relate to and appreciate, like when you're learning a hard concept in math and the teacher shares a practical example that clicks in your head and makes sense. I felt that I needed to put a face, a heart, and a soul to my food allergies that would allow others to relate to me. By humanizing myself and my situation, I would begin to build community. It was about being vulnerable and sharing, growing, and showing love for and supporting each other in order to *Be Healthy, Be Safe + Be Well™*. My parents had taught me that life is about service to others, and my changed mindset showed me that by humanizing my food allergies, I could achieve exactly that and gain so much more at the same time.

Humanizing begins with the ability to speak your truth, and speaking your truth begins with finding your voice by being vulnerable—slowly voicing your thoughts, dreams, and aspirations to others. Even if you do that just a little bit at a time, you will start to feel like you are breaking free from the chains and any past traumas that have bound you.

None of this work is easy, but it's incredibly rewarding! It took me a lot of dedicated time spent dreaming, whiteboarding, researching, and journaling everything I wanted to transform and how I wanted to (re)design my life. My 2008 incident lit the fire under my ass to make change because I finally believed that I deserved it. Because I *do* deserve it, and so do you.

Now it's time for you to use the tools you've put the blood, sweat, and tears into acquiring in the first parts of this book to be well. This final part of the *Three to Be™ Program* was extremely important to me, because it was about my well-being and giving back to humanity—and all of those people who have been there for me and watched over me my entire life.

Hilary Clinton once said, "Being human, we are imperfect. That's why we need each other. To catch each other when we falter. To encourage each other when we lose heart. Some may lead; others may follow; but none of us can go it alone. The changes we're working for are changes that we can only accomplish together".[67] She is right, because we all go through our own difficulties during our time on this Earth. To be there, support each other, empathize—that's what life is all about.

So, for one final time, I hope you enjoy the following chapters! Know that I am sending you light and love in your journey to be well.

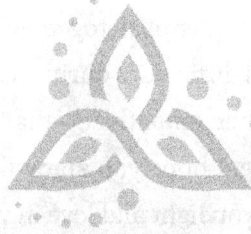

Stories of Wisdom on Learning to Advocate

What has been the greatest lesson(s) you learned from advocating about your food allergies?

Riya Miglani, Founder of the *Less Panic, More Peace* Podcast

"On a family vacation to Italy in 2018, my younger sister had two allergic reactions due to a chocolate croissant made with Nutella (which contains hazelnuts) and a coffee ice cream that was cross-contaminated with peanut butter ice cream. It was a really scary situation for all of us—my dad had to administer two EpiPens that week to counterbalance her allergic reactions! Seeing what she went through, I began advocating for my own food allergies and for other people with food allergies.

This was one of the main reasons that I created *Less Panic, More Peace: A Food Allergy Podcast*. On my podcast, I speak to others who are dealing with a similar allergy journey as what my sister and I have lived. It's always great to be able to relate to what they are going through, share stories, and talk about how we can all advocate for ourselves. I feel like I've given people with food allergies a foundation to help themselves and to help others who are new to life with allergies."

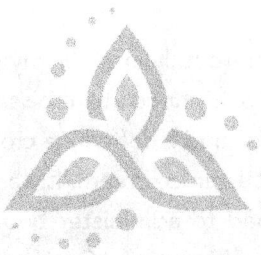

TEN

Learning to Advocate

"Womanhood taught me: staying silent about my story and struggle serves no one. I was given a voice, and I will share and speak up for women who feel voiceless."

— ALEX ELLE

LEARNINGS

In this chapter, we'll explore why staying silent about your food allergies does not serve you. You'll learn:

- Everyone has a voice that is beautiful, unique, and worthy.

- Speaking your truth is the key to becoming empowered.

- By advocating for your health, you can humanize your food allergies.

MY EARLY YEARS

For most of my life, I did not advocate for myself. I can't tell you how sad it was to reflect on this statement and put it in a book for the world to see! I don't wish that for anyone. Case in point: the donut situation in high school where I could have told my girlfriends that I had a nut allergy but chose to hide it because I was scared they wouldn't like me if I told them the truth. Another instance of shame was when someone found out about my food allergies and made me feel shitty about them, like what happened during my date with Hot Rod. Blimey!

My college years were no different. My parents were scared shitless at the thought of me eating on campus and trying to fit in with the crowd. As a freshman on the meal plan, mom and dad made me pinky swear to talk to someone in the food service program about my allergies. They threatened to do it for me if I didn't. During move-in day, I scoped out the vending machines in the lobby area to see what they had for sustenance. There were some snacky type of items that I could eat such as popcorn, but if I wanted to eat anything that resembled a real meal, it was a long trek to the dining hall from my dorm room. The effort had better be worth it!

Our dining hall had the usuals: salad bar, sandwich bar, hot meals, pizza, sodas/drinks, and a dessert station. Normally, I'd beeline it to the salad bar and stick with lettuce, tomatoes, cucumbers, with oil and vinegar for dressing, but the thought of eating salads for every meal for the next four years didn't appeal to me. So, I got in line behind my roommate and walked to the hot meals area, where she was loading some goulash stew into a bowl.

"Uh, do you know what's in this?" I quietly asked the dining staff person.

My roomie looked at me and said, "What, are you on some special diet or something?"

"Funny you should ask, biatch, because YES, I AM." Well, that's what I *wanted* to say, anyway. But the unempowered Sonia at the time gave out a nervous laugh and let the roomie move down the line.

"Do you think there are any nuts in this?" I asked the server again, poignantly but still very quietly.

"Nuts? No...well, I don't think so," he replied.

UGH! HOW CAN PEOPLE SERVE A DISH AND NOT KNOW WHAT'S

IN IT? #storyofmylife.

His answer unfortunately meant I needed to ask someone else. This brought more attention to myself, which I did not want on day one of college.

"Hey, what's your deal?" my roommate asked as she came back around to get me. I lied and told her that I didn't want to gain the "Freshman 15," so I wanted to know what was in the dish. She giggled and agreed it was a good plan not to gain weight…although she already had a dessert on her tray.

When she moved away again, I whispered to the server, "I can't have any nuts, so can you find out?"

Within minutes, I had held up the line and people were starting to go around me. The executive chef of the dining hall came out to find out what the questions were all about. Like a stealth hurricane about to unleash, I told the chef about my food allergies and that my parents were making me speak up; otherwise, I said, they'd come here and do it for me, and if he could tell me what I could eat and what I should stay away from, I'd forever be grateful. Sheesh!

"Wow, that's a lot in one sentence! But no problem—let's talk over here," he said.

This was a *huge* step for me! After all, I was keeping my word to my parents, *and* I had come clean with someone I didn't know in front of what felt like the entire freshman class. Hiding my food allergies and yet somehow getting by was second nature to me at this point. Going into college, I was so excited to be on my own! But I was also a bit scared of having to take care of my food allergies on my own. Not that I would ever say that to my parents. The chef was incredibly understanding and eager to learn more about how his staff could help.

Most of my life, I had been fighting a duality: one side was independent and didn't want someone speaking for me, and the other didn't want to bring attention to myself and liked having someone take care of me. Playing both sides was exhausting. Couldn't I just make up my mind? I did not tell my freshman year roommate or anyone else I met that year about my allergies, and that was a conscious decision. So, I worked the system in other ways:

- I quietly enlisted the executive chef and his staff for help whenever I ate in the dining hall. There was a time period where I didn't go there just to avoid the entire scene. That was a horrible decision! Thank goodness I did not end up with an eating disorder on top of everything else.

- I went home on weekends to eat and I talked my parents into dropping off home-cooked food as often as they could.

- I stocked up on unhealthy processed foods like pasta and ramen noodles for emergency situations where I needed to eat something that was "cleared of allergy items," yet none of those items were good for my overall health.

- I drank more and ate less.

- I was still popping a Benadryl® as a backup plan, if needed.

- I ate simple sandwiches (not bologna and cheese this time) I bought at the food trucks on campus because I knew that a turkey and cheese hoagie didn't have any nuts in it and therefore, I didn't need to share my information.

Do you see a theme here? My time in college was just more of the same as the years prior: not speaking up and just getting by. Which eventually caught up to me in 2008.

THE DAWN OF ADVOCATING FOR MYSELF

As a part of my transformation, I was now on a path to humanize my food allergies, and that process began with advocating for myself. With a changed mindset and having read copious self-help books after my 2008 incident, I hit a big realization: I had to start owning everything that was going on and speaking my truth. It was absolutely stupid to be afraid of or care about what anyone else thought about me or my food allergies. It only mattered what *I* thought. We don't learn that in school, yo! I think we should, because bullying starts young and leaves scars: physical, mental, spiritual, and emotional.

In 2008, it's not that I was lying about my food allergies the way I did in my youth. Everyone was just on a need-to-know basis. If I felt super-duper comfortable with you or I was forced into it, then you were in the know; otherwise, you were out. But now I needed to figure a few key things to begin advocating for myself:

- How did I need to feel in order to begin opening up about my food allergies?

- How could I start that conversation with others? What was my style going to be when I did this?

- Was anyone going to care?

- How would I handle the situation if someone then bullied me?

- How was I going to stop prioritizing what others thought and only prioritize what *I* thought?

I jotted down these and many more questions in my journal to begin figuring out my situation. One big thing was in my favor—hitting rock bottom in 2008 had flipped my script. It switched to a mindset that said, "Enough is enough—I cannot live this way anymore!" Even *one more day* of doing things the old way could have put me into the ground for good, or at least that's how I felt. To find my voice, I focused on two main areas: discovering that I had value as a beautiful and unique human, and starting to speak my truth.

DISCOVERING MY VALUE

Everyone provides something of value. (Yes, this is also on a yellow sticky on my bathroom mirror.) Advocating begins with believing in yourself. Believing in yourself means that you understand *you are a unique and valuable person*. It is an exercise in raising your self-esteem and knowing that you are worth the effort. When you know this in your soul, you can begin sharing this gloriousness with others, because others deserve to see and know the real you.

> **WHEN YOU FALL IN LOVE WITH YOURSELF, IT'S GAME OVER, BECAUSE YOU WILL BE UNSTOPPABLE!**

A beautiful passage from author Marianne Williamson sums up the place I was at this time in my life. "Our deepest fear is not that we are inadequate," she wrote. "Our deepest fear is that we are powerful beyond measure. It is our light, not our darkness that most frightens us. We ask ourselves, 'Who am I to be brilliant, gorgeous, talented, fabulous?' Actually, who are you not to be? You are a child of God. Your playing small does not serve the world".[68]

I should have had those words tattooed on my body. How many times had I played small because of my food allergies? How many times had I wanted to do things a different way, but hadn't had the guts to advocate for myself? "Too many," was the answer.

Playing small gets us nowhere! Please put that on a sticky note. Advocating for myself meant that I needed to see myself outside of my food allergies and I needed to see what value I held. My allergies had defined me for so long. No one really knew me without them, and I wanted people to get to know the real me. A part of me had always felt devalued as I was dealing with my disease, and that part had over-powered any sense of worth I had.

If I could articulate my value and really believe it, I could live it every day. I began writing down different areas of my life (in work and in play) where I believed I brought value to the world (and this was no time to be humble):

- **Kind soul:** I show kindness in everything I do.

- **Great friend:** I am the epitome of #rideordie! I go above and beyond for people I love, taking pride in remembering the small, personal things that make a difference to others.

- **Trust:** I am a confidant and great listener whom people trust and can openly talk to.

- **Committed:** I do what I say I am going to do, and I am deeply committed to everything I engage in.

- **Open-minded:** I listen and don't judge.

- **Humor:** I bring fun and funniness to tense situations.

- **Go Above and Beyond:** I create experiences in my relationships that evoke emotion and connectedness, such as hosting dinner parties.

- **Cooking:** I am a phenomenal cook who shows love to others by creating something beautiful and yummy for them.

- **Ideation:** I form new ways of looking at a problem.

- **Communication:** I am able to communicate with others easily and I can explain concepts that are technical and hard to understand in an easy way.

Writing all of this and more down on paper felt phenomenal! I would sooo date me! I felt so proud of myself! I kept saying "Yup! Uh-huh!" as I went through this exercise, because I whole-heartedly believed those words as I thought through the practical applications of each attribute. In believing them, I saw how unique I was because of all the beautiful qualities that make up me. I wasn't unique *just because* I had over 32 food allergies. Finally!

Now, I'm not perfect (nor do I try to be), but I knew that my qualities needed to be shared with the world so that I could continue to hone and improve them. Other people may have had the same skills, but they didn't do them or go about them the same way I did—my way was unique to me. I gabbed about this to my two besties, who laughed and just said, "Yes! Welcome to the party," as if they had known this the entire time. This realization gave me an exciting tingling feeling all over; it was like my entire being was screaming, "I have value and now I see it!" It was the loveliest of feelings, and I wanted everyone to have that feeling.

My therapist once told me that half the battle was just making the decision to advocate for myself and believing that I could do it, but belief in myself didn't just happen overnight for me. In fact, for years, my insecurity about my health situation led to insecurities in other areas of my life. But that's why working on myself every day—a little bit at a time!—was necessary to break free. The more I wrote down about what value I brought to the game called Life, the more I saw a beautiful human being I couldn't see before. Spending time on a daily basis working on myself has led me to be a better human to all those around me. I used this time to celebrate and give back to myself, and I still do this today.

SPEAKING MY TRUTH

When you are blocking or ignoring your truth, your body will tell you. My therapist and I discussed how pain and discomfort are natural repercussions of a life lived in the shadows. As children, we have someone taking care of us and watching over our well-being for the most part. But as adults, we can choose how we want to be; we can assert ourselves and claim our worth in the world. And doing that begins with noticing our body signals. Speaking your truth is about owning your voice and claiming your power.

> **"YOU ARE NOT DEFINED BY SOMEONE'S PARTIAL VIEW OF YOUR LIFE, YOUR STRENGTHS, OR YOUR HISTORY. THEIR INABILITY TO SEE OR APPRECIATE THE COMPLETE VERSION OF YOU ONLY LIMITS THEM, NOT YOU. STAND STRONG IN YOUR TRUTH AND YOUR PURPOSE AND CONTINUE BEING YOUR BADASS, UNAPOLOGETIC SELF".** [69]

This is a quote from the unapologetic speaker, author, and behaviorist Steve Maraboli, and it's definitely deserving of a yellow sticky note. What Steve is saying is that you are doing a disservice to yourself by putting so much emphasis on what other people's opinions of you are. Who the hell cares what someone else thinks of you? Where does it get you? In my case, it got me years of unhappiness and feeling chained.

Why did I care so much if my college roommate thought I was weird for having food allergies and asking questions about what was in the food? Because I wanted to be normal, and I defined "normal" as not having food allergies. But years later, with a changed mindset, I was able to see just how unique I was and how unique *everybody* is! There is not one person on this Earth who doesn't have something going on in their life that makes them feel insecure at times. So, I had to work on changing my mindset to not give a shit so much about others, but instead focus on giving a shit about what *I* thought and wanted. My allergies were my allergies—it's not like I prayed to God for them to come to me. It was just the hand that I was dealt, and it was a shitty hand. But now, I was working hard to play that hand in a different way. So why couldn't I say that out loud to everyone, because that *is* my truth? Well, I guess I just did.

In order to start speaking my truth, I went into research mode again. After having read many books about the human psyche and talking through all of this in partnership with my therapist, I identified the following five steps to take:

Step One: Noticing Body Signals. I observed when my body had sensations that felt good or bad. For example, if someone raised their voice with me, I would get a negative tingly feeling. Just the opposite happened if I was excited about something: I'd get a positive tingly feeling. Then I thought about the difference between those two scenarios and reactions. You get what I'm staying—starting to notice the sensations in your body and the context in which they appear is the key.

I began immediately writing down whenever I felt negative tingling and tried to pinpoint exactly what had caused that feeling. In my mind, I made a mental note of the situation—whether it was a tone of voice, a raised voice, or an actual person. Then if it happened again, I immediately would breathe for ten seconds to calm down before managing my reaction to it/them. This is so hard to do! But with practice, it will come.

Step Two: Determining my Role. Nothing is ever one-sided, so this step was about determining what role I was playing in my own misery. For example, was I enabling others? This was about exploring my role in each of these situations and then documenting why I felt that it was wrong and identifying a new action and result. In taking responsibility for myself, I became the leader of my life rather than the follower, in the process also letting go of my victim mentality.

I thought through situations where I felt small or slighted, dissected them truthfully, and wrote down how I wanted to change each one. I cross-referenced them against situations where my body signals were negative and began to pinpoint how I had reacted in that situation and how I wanted to react in the future. The next time the same situation came up, I took my ten-second peace-out time and then would try a different response. Back to the example of my college roomie: it was on me to tell her the truth about my food allergies, because we were about to share a room for the next year and food definitely would be involved. It wasn't fair for her to be in the dark, and I didn't need to pay it any mind if she thought I was weird. I had to own it, and that was that.

Step Three: Laying Down Boundaries. Author Mark Mansen states, "Healthy personal boundaries = taking responsibility for your own actions and emotions while *not* taking responsibility for the actions or emotions of others".[70] Not setting healthy boundaries means we tend to spend our time and energy doing what *others* want us to do over what *we* want to do, which leads to frustration and depression because we feel unfulfilled or lost. But there are lessons in everything, from listening to your intuition to creating boundaries around your time and life, valuing your own ideas, and/or asserting yourself. You can also learn from saying "no" and putting up a boundary rather than always saying "yes" and appeasing others. In taking this step, I was moving from playing a reactive role to laying down healthy boundaries for myself through conscious action, growth, and personal responsibility.

In documenting in this process, I learned that I had never been comfortable speaking my truth about my food allergies because I was never direct about what I wanted or didn't want. Note: that's a boundary. I also had not made my safe-care a priority before this process. That's also a boundary. Allowing others to make me feel a certain way and not speaking up for myself? Yup—boundary. I had major passive-aggressive behavior going on in my life!

So, like a madwoman strategizing, I began countering every unhealthy boundary with a positive one by writing "When X situation happens, now you will do Y" and putting those words into practice. For example, I would notice when someone invaded my boundaries, because my body would get that bad, tingly feeling. The difference? Now I spoke up by telling the person that they had not taken my feelings into account and that I needed them to—and then I would state my feelings. In other words, I called out the negative action in an unthreatening way and tried to get a positive reaction out of it. And I did this with kindness and my own style because I didn't want to treat someone badly, even if I had felt they had treated me that way.

It's important to note that this was more about me working the steps to speak my truth than trying to convince someone to change their shitty behavior.

Step Four: Being Self Aware. Ah, self-awareness, you beautiful beast, you!

I've always been so hard on myself—harder than my teachers or bosses have ever been—because I was always trying to strive for some idea of perfection. In this process, I learned that it's not about perfection, it's about progress and the journey. That is still on a sticky note!

Self-awareness was about my ability to notice my feelings, physical sensations, reactions, habits, behaviors, and thoughts. I had to move the negative inner critic that had held me down for years, telling me that I wasn't capable or that I would do it wrong. That inner critic gave me seemingly sound reasons why I should keep my mouth shut, because in that situation, fear was doing its job. It was trying to protect "me" by keeping me safe in a bubble, away from the unknown and further hurt. That's called a "cognitive distortion," and it was warping how I saw things, including myself. It was something I immediately needed to change to be free.

So, every time I wanted to use my voice but my inner critic came out and told me "You shouldn't/couldn't/wouldn't," I began clicking my inner critic the hell out of the way, because that vocabulary no longer served me. Being self-aware that this was happening was the key to hearing the click that went off in my head anytime my negative inner critic came out.

Step Five: Courageously Speaking my Truth. It was time to actually put those first four steps into practice! I needed to start believing and dreaming about being free from past trauma related to my food allergies. My language was changing: I was beginning to talk and act like speaking my truth was going to happen! But I wanted to

determine what my communication style was in order to advocate
for myself.

I decided that I wanted my voice to be reflective of the unique and
beautiful parts of me that were inside waiting to get out, so I wrote in my
journal what that looked like. It was going to be kind, yet direct; sweet
and empowered; empathetic to the person I was dealing with; and all
executed with the flavor of my fun personality. I wanted to speak my
truth with a smile on my face even in the face of adversity. On a daily
basis, I practiced expressing my feelings in real-life situations before
asking for what I wanted. This helped me to connect with other people
as well as communicate the importance of my request.

HOW YOU CAN ADVOCATE FOR YOURSELF

My wish for you is that you do all things in life with love. If you
do not give yourself love, kindness, and forgiveness, then you have no
love, kindness, and forgiveness to give to others. Most of the exercises
in the *Three to Be™ Program* will force you to take a deep, hard look
within at what is going on in your health and your life that is or is not
serving you. During these exercises, it's important to be completely
transparent and honest with yourself. Know that there is no wrong
answer. If there are things you want to change for the better, you
can set that desire in your mind and begin to achieve it by taking
microsteps today.

Step One: Feeling the Pain and Growing from It. Do not
get to the point of hitting rock bottom to begin your transformation!
Begin now by digging deep, strategizing, and journaling about the
following questions:

• What is your truth as it relates to your health and well-being?
  Create a statement around this and write it in your journal.

- Are you openly speaking that truth or hiding it from the world? If you're hiding, go deeper and ask yourself exactly why that's happening. Write down exact situations where you did not speak up and advocate for yourself and counter those with ways to change that behavior in the future.

- Write down a list of what is holding you back from freeing yourself and living the life you want, food allergies and all. What are you scared of?

As you begin to answer these questions, more will pop into your head. All of them will help you pinpoint exactly what is holding you back from hitting your North Star. Once you begin to understand what fears hold you back, you can stare them in the eyes and chip away at them.

Step Two: Seeing Your Value. Begin by writing down the top 10 areas in which you bring value to the world. You *must* write down 10...and you can keep going! If you cannot think of any, then do this exercise along with someone from your support team. We can be our own worst critics; at times, those who love us unconditionally can see more about our life from afar than we can while living it.

Look at this list every day. I want you to feel great about this list, because it's unique to you! Only *you* can bring that special flavor of differentiation to the world. The way you are committed to doing things will absolutely be different than the way anyone else is committed, even if they're committed to the same things.

Step Three: Creating Steps to Advocacy. Start writing down detailed ideas about how you can improve the way you speak up for yourself and your food allergies. Is there an inner critic in your head that is always being Negative Nelly and stopping you from speaking up?

Do you have the verbiage to use when you *do* speak up? Is it assertive and complimentary to you, or is it self-deprecating? When you analyze this information, you'll begin to see negative behaviors, patterns, and habits.

Also, during this process, surround yourself with people from your support team who have a beautiful sense of self and are advocates. Whether you know them personally or follow them online, they will be a great inspiration to you. Ask them how they began advocating for themselves to get tips.

Self-advocacy leads to independence, which means being free from past trauma and having the ability to finally take responsibility and ownership for yourself.

THE NET NET

A quick reminder that when you fall in love with yourself, it's game over, because you will be unstoppable! By using these techniques and taking microsteps daily, I finally learned how to advocate for and love myself. I went from:

- Allowing others to speak for me —► Using my own voice.

- Caring what others thought about me —► Caring about what I thought about myself.

- Letting my inner critic rule —► Using informed judgment and in some cases my gut feelings.

- Not having boundaries/having unhealthy boundaries —► Setting up healthy boundaries.

- Overanalyzing everything —► Doing just the right amount of analysis to keep myself healthy and safe.

- Downplaying and hiding my food allergies —▶ Talking openly and proactively about my food allergies to my support team, and to the world.

Through this work, I learned a lot about what was holding me back and how I could easily change those negatives into positive, healthy behaviors, patterns, and/or habits. When I took the time to really work this out, I realized that the answer had always been right there in front of me! I finally saw myself as a cool person who brought a tremendous amount of goodness to the world, goodness that I wanted to share with everyone! It was freeing to feel this way.

The biggest realization I had was that my voice was worthy. And that the more I used it, the more I could and would transform into a beautiful human who was open to anything that might come my way. I was confident that I could deal with it all, whether it was health-related or something else. Realizing all of this gave me the power and courage I had been seeking for so many years to be prepared for whatever was to come.

Everyone deserves a life that is bright with potential. I had always prided myself on the fact that my Indian culture is all about honor and respect, yet I had to learn the hard way to honor and respect *myself* first before I could give honor and respect to others. Recognizing what was holding me back was key to finding the courage to advocate for myself. Finding my voice and starting to consistently use it was a gargantuan step for me. It's not that I never had a voice—I did! But I had to look deep down and find the courage to believe in it and what it could be used for. Post 2008, advocating meant consistently speaking up for myself in a way I never had before. And it also meant using my voice to help others who were struggling to find theirs.

All of the years prior to 2008, I had been looking at everything the wrong way: I was only looking at myself. When I turned around that view to focus externally and started seeing others as allies and people who could benefit from my knowledge—and started talking to them about my situation—then I believed that good would prevail and they would care enough to help me if I ever needed their help.

Being free from your food allergies means that you accept them, you accept yourself, and you will lead your best possible life with or without them. I set out to be a beacon of hope to many others in my same situation who were looking for other methods to cope with their situations.

So, where do we go from here? In 2008, when my testing clocked in at over 32 food allergies, I began thinking about how to use my voice and explain those allergies to someone without the explanation it taking hours on end. I didn't want to rattle off my allergies and make a server frantically try to keep up. I also needed a way to humanize my food allergy list so that someone could associate me with the allergies. And it all probably needed to be written down!

I embarked upon creating a tool that I could use to open doorways and advocate for myself. This tool was not to be a crutch—rather, it was something that would make my situation easy to understand, informative, and fun! Thus, the idea of my super cool food allergy card was born.

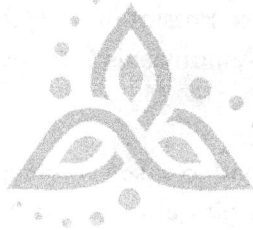

Stories of Wisdom on Designing a Food Allergy Card

How can tools like food allergy cards help someone with allergies be safe and become empowered?

Eleanor Garrow-Holding, President and Chief Executive Officer of the Food Allergy & Anaphylaxis Connection Team

"In 2004, my 19-month-old son Thomas was diagnosed with life-threatening food allergies after an anaphylactic reaction to pecans at a family birthday party. Although there were many support groups for families dealing with food allergies in Chicago and the suburbs, there were none where we lived. From that day on, I started educating myself and my family on everything related to food allergies and anaphylaxis. Reading labels every time we purchased products and calling manufacturers to ask about cross-contact or if the product had been manufactured on shared lines or in the same facility became our new norm. My mom—a nurse—was a great support, as were other parents.

Since I didn't have a local group to participate in, I started PO-CHA of Will County (Parents of Children Having Allergies). Parents loved the in-person meetings and socialization. It was great to meet other families who shared the same life experiences.

I knew I could not let Thomas's food allergies define him or hold us back from living life. I was not going to let fear take over, nor was I going to allow anyone to instill fear in us! Living with food allergies is manageable. I taught Thomas how to advocate for himself at a young age, and he has always been his own best advocate. I am so proud of him! My best advice, it is especially important to not lose sight of your family members who are not allergic. Food allergies affect the entire family, including siblings. Lastly, know that you are not alone—support is there for you and your family."

ELEVEN

Designing a Food Allergy Card

> "Your value will be not what you know; it will be what you share."
>
> — GINNI ROMETTY

LEARNINGS

In this chapter, we'll explore tools to have in your arsenal that will empower you and help you to advocate about your food allergies. You'll learn:

- A food allergy card allows you to start a conversation.

- Your card will be rooted with intention.

- In sharing your card, you will be educating others and humanizing food allergies.

MY EARLY YEARS

When I was a teenager, my mom and her best friend became first-time entrepreneurs and started a restaurant. It was amazing to see women in my life bring this to life! They even had a beautiful full-page article written up about them in *The Philadelphia Inquirer*'s dining section. My cousin and I got roped into working there as servers after school, but we got paid and ate an unlimited supply of their delicious food, so somehow it evened out.

During the time I worked there, I never served anyone who had food allergies, or at least no one ever verbalized to me that they did. Plenty of people had food preferences like "Not too spicy!" or "I hate cilantro." But no one outwardly voiced their food restrictions, and I never asked since I was in my hiding phase. Also, I figured if someone really couldn't eat a food item, they would speak up, like my parents did when *we* went out to eat and servers took our orders.

One day, I waited on a customer who ordered a curry that had heavy cream in the base. Almost instantly after eating it he ran to the men's room, stating that he didn't feel well after he returned. My mom came out from the kitchen and spoke to him about every ingredient in the dish and mentioned "heavy cream," and then he stopped her stating he had issues with dairy. Trust me, my mama ain't no fool—she asked if it was an allergy and if he had told his server (in this case, me) about his allergy. The customer said it was not a food allergy and he had not said anything because he hadn't thought there was dairy in Indian curries. He ended up apologizing and said he loved the food and would be back again, but to eat a curry made without dairy.

Throughout this exchange, teenage me was sitting in the corner eavesdropping and sweating bullets. Had I made someone sick? Then I had to listen to my mother lecturing me about the situation all the way home. "Why would he not say anything, especially if dairy gives him diarrhea? And to act like my *curry* was the problem? Ha! He should see your allergist!"

During our family dinner that night, the conversation somehow became about me and how I shouldn't be like *that guy.* "You have so many allergies. Who can remember? You have to start opening your mouth and telling people so they can write it down," was the gist of the message from my mom.

Why did my mother always have to be right??? I pooh-poohed her suggestion back then because I was not about to publicize my food issues on paper, but she was certainly foreshadowing a time when this would come back to bite me.

After my 2008 incident, I realized that I needed a new way to communicate—I couldn't just rattle off over 32 items to a server who surely wasn't going to remember any of them. I needed a food allergy card.

WHY RESTAURANTS WANT A FOOD ALLERGY CARD

Given my family's background in the restaurant industry and as a major foodie who loves the dining out experience, I've always been personally invested in the success of restaurants. As a part of my transformation, I wanted to help them help people like me. I set out to understand how we could begin to bridge the gap between restaurants and the food allergy community in a new way.

The 2016 Restaurant Legislation toolkit from the Food Allergy Research & Education Organization (FARE) details research that suggests that more than half of fatal food allergy reactions are triggered by food consumed outside the home[71].

- "According to a survey by the National Restaurant Association, some 87% of restaurants believe food allergies are extremely important and expect increased attention to it, yet 43% concede they do not train their staff on food allergens".[72]

- "Researchers at Auburn University surveyed 110 restaurant managerial staff in the U.S. from both independent and chain restaurants to investigate the levels of awareness and preparedness related to serving customers with food allergies. Among their findings, nearly 22% of participants indicated food allergy reactions had occurred at their restaurants in the past year. Also, even though 80% of participants indicated they had received training about food allergies, there were wide gaps in knowledge about food allergies. For example, about 40% believed that simply removing a food allergen from a plated meal could prevent an allergic reaction".[73]

· "Currently, the revenue lost from food allergy families avoiding restaurant dining is estimated at $45 million each week—more than $2 billion annually".[74]

· "The global food market for those with food allergies is projected to exceed $24.8 billion by 2020".[75]

· "The multiplier effect of more than 15 million Americans on restaurant patronage can have a substantial impact on those establishments accommodating the food allergy customer".[76]

Designed to make it safer for individuals with food allergies to dine in restaurants, state laws may include provisions like notices on menus asking patrons to inform the server about any food allergies, food allergy training for restaurant managers, and procedures to inform customers, upon request, of the presence of major food allergens in menu items. "Thus far, California, Illinois, Massachusetts, Maryland, Michigan, Rhode Island, Virginia, and St. Paul, Minnesota all have enacted laws to improve food allergy safety and awareness in restaurants".[77]

WOWZA! As I already knew, it's not like those of us with food allergies don't want to eat out. It's that the trust factor is not there because the education, laws, and processes and procedures are not in place across the industry. And dare I say, the empathy is not there, either. We have a long way to go, but we can do it! I felt that a tool like a food allergy card that everyone in the restaurant who serviced me could look at as they made my food would drastically help them *and* me. The data certainly shows that the use case is there! So, I began my part to help move this partnership along.

WHY I NEEDED A FOOD ALLERGY CARD

I'm the person who creates a grocery list on paper every week. I heavily use Evernote on my computer for tasks and I use Siri to remind myself of things as they pop into my head. And as you know, I am a whiteboarding and journaling maniac! Go figure how someone as organized and analytical as me *didn't* carry a food allergy card. Even though I had my 32 plus food allergies memorized in my own head, there was no way I could expect anyone else to remember them. I felt that it was my responsibility to remind others and provide some easy way for them to keep track of my litany of allergies whenever I was in a dining situation.

My aha moment came when I was filling out paperwork at each new doctor's office in the months following my anaphylaxis incident in 2008. In that paperwork, I had to list any allergies to food and/or medications. In the process of writing my allergies down for what felt like a gazillion times, I thought it would be much easier if I could just hand them a card or even email them a digital file with this information.

Thanks to all of the hard work I had done to deconstruct myself, I felt that my card had to consist of more than just a written list of items—it had to have meaning and purpose, and it had to be a vehicle I could use in working toward my North Star. It had to reflect the new me who was done with self-sabotaging and all about empowered advocacy. I wasn't going to go to a restaurant for a meal and just say, "Here's my list—deal with it!" Rather, I was on a path to humanize the conversation around my food allergies by truly connecting with other people, who could then offer a helping hand when needed.

As part of my job, one of the first things I hand out when I meet someone new is my business card. So, I began thinking about my food allergy card like my new business card, one that provided my pertinent information within the context of dining.

DESIGNING MY FOOD ALLERGY CARD

My design process began by ideating possibilities of what my food allergy card could be, and then creating it, testing it, and utilizing it as a tool for advocacy. This card going to have many benefits for me, including:

- It would clearly state my list of allergies so that restaurant staff and chefs wouldn't have to remember them.

- It would allow restaurant staff to cross-reference my allergies with ingredients in their dishes.

- It would allow me to begin a conversation around my food allergies with ease and ask lots of questions.

- It would help me dine out safely and enjoy an allergy-friendly meal.

To begin bringing my card to life, I enlisted help from a few folks on my support team, including my dear friend and acclaimed chef Scott Howard. We had met through mutual friends before the opening of his restaurant Five in the Hotel Shattuck in Berkeley, California, and we had become fast friends for life. Scott is an amazing chef and wonderful human being who took immediate interest in my food allergy situation.

"Damn, girl. How're you surviving?" he said with a southern drawl when I first met him. He was interested in how I ate at restaurants given that he has two children of his own and had dealt with food allergies in their schools. We discussed my notion of writing it all down in a card format to make it easier for the restaurant staff to cook for me.

"Great idea! Just give me the card when you're done, and I'll make sure we keep it in the restaurant," he said.

"What are you gonna do with it? Is it gonna sit in your office?" I replied.

"I'm gonna make sure my guys in the kitchen know about this so that no one messes up your dishes when you come in. And I'll keep it in the office so you can still eat if I'm not there. Trust me, I don't want you dying in my restaurant!" he said.

True dat, Chef Howard! So, this was interesting—he was going to keep my upcoming food allergy card in his office so that the staff could know my list of allergies whenever I came in. That was even better than I had expected!

In order to create a tool like a food allergy card, I first needed to understand how restaurants deal with food restrictions, what information should go on my card, and how the two would connect. I wrote down an exhaustive list of questions on my whiteboard and worked with various people in the restaurant industry (including my parents) to get to the answers.

- What is a restaurant's process from the front of the house to the back of the house when relaying dietary restrictions?

- How does that information get translated from person to person and eventually to the chef making my meal?

- How would a restaurant utilize a food allergy card?

- What training, if any, does restaurant staff have on food allergies?

- How trained is the waitstaff about the ingredients in their dishes?

- How can I help educate restaurants about food allergies and my situation?

I began sketching a 360-degree picture of what it would be like to feed me in a restaurant. The same process could be used (and would be much easier to use) when eating at someone's house, because a home cook is not dealing with hundreds of diners at the same time. Empathy was top of mind, as I really wanted to understand what a restaurant goes through when serving someone like me. Then in return and in partnership, I could help them with how to provide me with a wonderful dining experience. Talk about a win-win situation!

I also discussed all of this with my dear friend and chef Alexander Ong at Betelnut Restaurant in San Francisco. I absolutely *love* spicy Asian food, but it was always in the no-no category when eating out. He talked to me about cleaning procedures for cross-contamination, and how he substituted ingredients in the Asian foods he was cooking for me. I continued to talk to other chefs in the Bay Area and learned a tremendous amount of information about how restaurants dealt with food allergies (or not). In 2009, Bill S. 2701 was passed, requiring restaurants to "...take a few straightforward precautions in order to ensure the safety of their diners with food allergies. Signed into law last month (2009), the bill goes (went) into effect April 15, 2010".[78] But this was only in the state of Massachusetts. The net net is that it still was and still *is* up to each restaurant to either accommodate or not accommodate a customer with dietary restrictions such as food allergies. For the restaurants that choose to accommodate diners with dietary restrictions, I learned how individualized the process was given that each restaurant's depth of information regarding food allergies varied so greatly.

If you've ever been out to eat, you know that several people could be interacting with you during your experience: the owner, host, bartender, server, supplemental waitstaff, chef, pastry chef, and bus crew. Trying to keep information constant and consistent between all of these people is a chore. That was another reason why I felt that a food allergy card could help their process while it helped me.

Depending on the size of the restaurant, servers typically write down orders and put that ticket into a system or hand the ticket to the kitchen staff. I felt that having an allergy card attached to that information would make it stand out. Another thing I learned was that there was no food allergy training in culinary school (at least, not at that time), nor did restaurants generally provide any training on food allergies. This meant I would need to ask copious amounts of questions to make sure I understood what ingredients were in dishes. I would also have to state clearly on my card what I could not eat. I've always said, when you have severe food allergies, it's like you gain a Ph.D. in food science! For example, I am allergic to almonds, which also means I cannot have almond oil, almond flour, or almond butter! I once was served a dessert made with almond flour because the server thought I only could not have almonds themselves. D'oh!

Serving people with food allergies is not an easy process for anyone involved. That's why I felt that the more I learned from restaurant staff, the safer I could keep myself. After all, I was the one making the conscious decision to eat out.

Taking into account all that I had learned from the restaurant industry, I made some key design choices for my pending allergy card:

- The design needed to be unique to me—something that attracted attention in a good way and made the recipient feel something.

- The information must be laid out in a way that was easy to understand.

- It must be small enough to fit into my clutch or back pocket, yet large enough to read.

- Choosing the right template, font size, and font style was key.

- It needed to list emergency numbers.

I emailed a black-and-white version to my mother, who said, "If something happens to you, how would someone know to call me or your father?" OMG, this woman is a psychic! She was right. I added the names of both of my parents and their mobile phone numbers to the right of 911 so that they were in order of importance. I also got all fancy and hired a graphic designer to create a logo for my name so that it would stand out on my card and make it look cool.

After playing with the layout a million times and running it by Chef Howard and Chef Ong and others on my support teams and at restaurants, I had a local printer print it on cardstock. I felt incredibly accomplished—I was owning my allergies and speaking my truth! Like a beast, I was ready to unleash my new concept into the restaurant world and conduct some testing.

GAINING INSIGHTS FROM TESTING MY CARD

I went back to Chef Howard's restaurant, where we had agreed to do a test with his own staff without their knowledge. (Hee, hee!) We sat at a table and one of his servers came to wait on us. I stated that I had some severe food allergies that the kitchen needed to know about and handed her the card.

As she looked at it, her eyes popped out of her head like Michael Keaton in the 1988 film *Beetlejuice*. "Whoa, these are a lot of food allergies! Chef, what do you want me to do with this?" That was the first sign of progress and validated what the process would be like.

"Yes, Chef, what would you like to do with my card?" I asked cloyingly. Chef went into the kitchen with the server and my card. When he came back, he said he had shown it to the staff and they had discussed my order. "What did they say?" I asked with excitement.

"They asked me who the three-headed monster was in our dining room."

Whaat??? My heart sank. They probably pictured a sad, pathetic girl with big boils or something. I pictured them making fun of me in the kitchen while having the arduous task of cooking something for me that wouldn't kill me, all because their boss told them to.

"Hey, don't be down! Guys can be jerks. This is great data for you, though," Chef said. And you know what? He was absolutely right!

I conducted this same test with ten other restaurants in San Francisco. At some, I knew the owner, but I didn't at most of them. At all of the restaurants, I gained so many data points that would help me tweak my card into its final form! As some of the feedback was consistent across the restaurants, I bucketed feedback into three areas:

behavioral, process, and education. Then I used those categories to further refine my card.

Step One: Creating an Easy Layout. Overall, there was some difficulty reading all of the information on my card because there was so darn much of it. I remedied that by increasing the font size and laying out my allergies in groupings such as Nuts, Fish, and Medications. (My doctors gave me the feedback that I needed to include my medication allergies on the card, because, yes...I also have medication allergies!) Lord have mercy! Another tweak I made was to put my allergic items into alphabetical order within their groupings to help the information flow better. Another interesting find was that most restaurant staff had never seen a card like mine nor a list so long, so they weren't quite sure what to do with it. More on that in the next few steps.

Step Two: Beginning a Conversation. Almost 100 percent of the servers I spoke to did not know the difference between a peanut, a tree nut, and a pine nut. I had a lot of work ahead of me. Some big issues required much partnership with the restaurant owners and chefs in this area, including how the waitstaff "viewed" my card, as there were some derogatory statements when it was first presented. When they go low, we go high! I took the high road on that and chose to ignore those comments, because my safety was the top-most priority, not my feelings. Using the tool set I described in "Chapter 10: Learning to Advocate," I used my voice and didn't lose control.

I reminded myself that I could control absolutely nothing in this process except my own choices and decisions. In the past, I would have felt disdain toward anyone who didn't know that a pine nut was a seed and not the same thing as a peanut. But my intention was not to berate waitstaff who had never learned about any of this to begin with—my intention was to utilize my card to begin a conversation with the waitstaff and see if they could help me maneuver eating at a restaurant safely. Conversations in person are key! And it was on me to be my own advocate.

Step Three: Helping Educate Staff. As I was ordering food, I would always educate the waitstaff by saying things like this: "Pine nuts are okay because they are a seed. Sesame is also okay for me, because it's also a seed and I am not allergic to seeds. But peanuts are a NO, because they are not a seed and I am severely allergic to them." Through asking probing questions with a sweet demeanor, I used my lifetime of education and knowledge of food allergies and began sharing it. It felt really great to do this! I made so many new friends who came to know me because of my card.

I also offered to provide more education to staff; some chefs then invited me to come to their pre-service meeting to briefly speak about food allergies. This was an amazing opportunity to humanize my food allergies.

Step Four: Aligning My Card with the Dining Process. From the moment my card left my hand, food was constantly spilled on it, which at times made the black ink run. I remedied this by laminating the card—that made it easy to wipe spills and fingerprints away, plus then line cooks could look it at while cooking my meal. (The flimsy unlaminated card didn't hold up well on the line.) This was a key point, because as tickets came in from servers, that meant that my card stood out to everyone making my meal!

Another data point was that my card also was not passed along to every person who touched my meal, meaning sometimes the head chef did not even see my card. Once again, it was on me to have an in-depth conversation with the server and then ask questions about what had happened in the kitchen when they brought my food out. For example, had the head chef personally made my meal? If so, did they have my card in front of them while making the dish? Had anyone else contributed to my dish in addition to the chef? Asking these questions when my food was brought out to me was my way of double-checking that things were copacetic.

Step Five: Showing Empathy to All Beings. I know that no one *needs* to help me. Doing so should be their choice, and I was comfortable understanding that because I had worked through caring about what other people thought. (Woot-woot for me for learning about and changing my own negative behaviors!) If any negative energy came from anyone I shared my food allergy card with, I wanted to understand it so that I could possibly help. Or I got up and left. I wasn't about to spend so much (hard-earned!) time transforming just to possibly put myself in harm's way.

For example, when Chef Howard's kitchen staff asked, "Who's the three-headed monster in the dining room?" I showed them who I was by sashaying into the kitchen with a smile on my face as I shook the hand of every person and let them know how grateful I was that they were using my allergy card to make me a safe meal. Talk about having a bunch of guys eating out of your hand! Then the magic started as one person asked me questions about my food allergies and another told me his daughter had a dairy allergy. Yay for empathy! I made this a regular thing if the chef or restaurant allowed it—I would peek into the kitchen and thank the staff, leaving with new friends and the hope that they would help another person like me in the future.

Over the last decade, I've worked with countless restaurants to understand how food allergy information is translated in a workflow, from the onset of the reservation to the end of the meal. Exchanging information with staff, giving them tips, and going through mock scenarios all helps restaurants better accommodate someone like me. Yes, technology can help throughout this process, but so much of it is about making human connections!

The final piece of feedback I received would later become my signature thang. It was something I had heard from some celebrity chefs as I attended several high-profile food and wine festivals around the country. Food and wine events typically were not my scene—any type of event where chefs are making bites in bulk to feed the masses is a bad place for someone with food allergies. It can be chaotic as guests fight to grab a picture with their favorite celebrity chef and snag a plate of whatever they are serving! Within that chaos, there's not much time for a lengthy discussion about ingredients in a dish. But I was still in the process of gathering feedback from those within the food service industry, so these types of events seemed to be a good place to test my card.

Many chefs had the same eye-popping *Beetlejuice* moment when they saw my card at their table in a Grand Tasting, and carefully ran down my list to confirm if I could eat their bite or not.

"It would be cool if you put your picture on your card. You know, so the kitchen knows who you are," was the sentiment from interested parties about my story on carrying my allergy card.

I loved that idea! It was another step toward humanizing my food allergies.

Selecting the picture for my card was a big deal, because it represented the key intersection of me, my allergies, and my dish for whomever was going to cook for me. I needed to entice someone to find out more about me and ask questions, and I wanted my card to leave a lasting impression. It had to wow at first sight! In true form, I went one step further and hired a professional photographer to take my picture. Why the hell not, right? Once we had gotten the glamour shot I wanted, I played around with different sizes on either the front or back of the card. I even had friends on my support team vote on which picture to use.

All of this research, talking to people, testing, getting feedback, and tweaking led me to this super coolio food allergy card. It is direct and to the point; it's cute, it's sassy, and it's me.

SONIA HUNT   FOOD ALLERGIES

PEANUTS + TREE NUTS

- Almonds (+ Oil, Flour, Butter)
- Brazil Nuts (+ Oil, Flour, Butter)
- Cashews (+ Oil, Flour, Butter)
- Chestnuts (+ Oil, Flour, Butter)
- Hazelnuts (+ Oil, Flour, Butter)
- Peanuts (+ Oil, Flour, Butter)
- Pecans (+ Oil, Flour, Butter)
- Pistachios (+ Oil, Flour, Butter)
- Walnuts (+ Oil, Flour, Butter)

OTHER FOODS

- Avocado (+Oil, Butter)
- Banana
- Buckwheat
- Cantaloupe
- Celery
- Corn
- Honeydew
- Halibut
- Rye
- Sesame
- Soybean
- Tomato

MEDICATIONS

- Erythromycin
- Keflex
- Penicillin

911 | Mom (123) 555-0000 | Dad (123) 555-1111

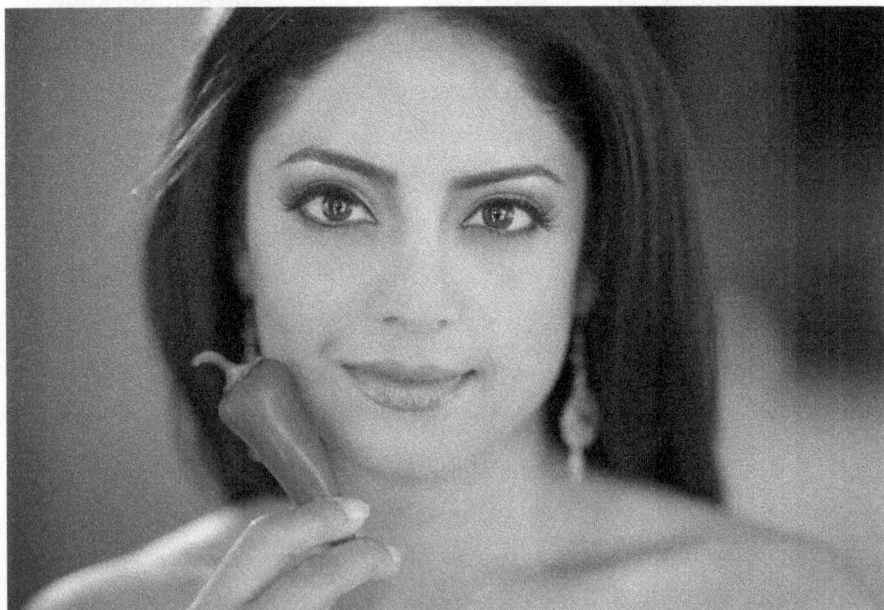

I printed hundreds of copies of my new food allergy card and placed them in every single purse, clutch, gym bag, shopping bag, suitcase, and laptop bag that I owned. I also placed some around my house next to the multiple EpiPen® Auto Injectors I keep seeing as the two go hand in hand. But I really I wanted to rent an airplane and throw them out into the sky! To take my advocacy to another level, I also gave copies to friends on my support team. Several restaurant chefs and owners also asked for a copy for them to keep on file. Breakthroughs were happening on all levels!

Looking back, I couldn't believe I hadn't carried around a card like this before! I mean, how the hell had everyone around me been operating? The energy I felt when I got feedback like "Sonia, I love this card! It's amazing! I wish everyone who has food allergies carried one!" made me feel like I was on fire, especially because it was coming from restaurant staff. I had a visceral feeling that I was on to something great. My card opened doors to real human connections and conversations because I had piqued people's interest and they wanted to know more and learn more, plus they felt that I had just made their job easier. And this, my friends, was a foundational tool for keeping myself healthy, safe, and well.

HOW YOU CAN DESIGN YOUR FOOD ALLERGY CARD

If you don't have a food allergy card, no worries! I've made it super easy for you.

Step One: Use a Template. At the back of this book, you'll find a Resources section with a pre-formatted, pop-out food allergy card. Just fill it out, and *voilà*! You have a card you can begin using today! I do recommend taking that card to your local printer and asking them to laminate it, as many people may be touching your card in a kitchen.

Step Two: Design your Own. Your food allergy card is one of the greatest, most personalized tools for advocacy you can have. Use a tool like Microsoft PowerPoint or Adobe Photoshop to create something unique that showcases your own style. You should feel comfortable with the information you put on the card as others will see it, but I recommend including the following:

- Your name (you'd be surprised at how many people forget this)

- Emergency phone numbers: 911 and then the mobile numbers for your parents and/or other emergency contacts

- Your food allergy list

- Your medication allergies (if any)

- Disclaimers and/other important information (i.e., you carry an EpiPen®)

Regarding disclaimers, I love the one that FARE (Food Allergy Research & Education) has on their website! It reads:

"Please make sure that my food does not contain any of the ingredients on the front of this card and that any utensils and equipment used to prepare my meal—as well as prep surfaces—are fully cleaned immediately before using. THANK YOU for your help".[79]

You can use that verbatim on your card, or you can create your own statement. It's important to also talk to the staff at a restaurant and ask questions about their prep areas, surfaces, etc. For example, because I have an avocado allergy, when eating sushi, I make sure to not only tell the server about my allergy, but I ask them to tell the chef to cut my sushi with a clean knife and clean cutting board. If they cannot accommodate me, they must tell me they cannot. So, conversations around these disclaimers will reveal a lot of information about what the restaurant's processes are. I also have kept track of all of this information in a personal database for my own use. You knew I would, right?

THE NET NET

My food allergy card has single-handedly saved my life multiple times. I have used this card all over the world, even translating it into different languages to use when I travel. It is always with me! I never leave home without it. I even stopped giving out my business card and began handing out my food allergy card instead. The people who have seen my card have been so grateful that I took the time and effort to help them help me. Servers and staff in restaurants see my card and say, "Oh, yeah, I remember you! I helped you before. I love your card! I wish everyone carried one."

It's important to note that I have never looked at or used my food allergy card as a crutch. Instead, it is a tool in my arsenal (along with my other tools) that I have used to set myself free of all of the trauma in my past life around my food allergies.

When it comes to advocating for myself, carrying a food allergy card has been one huge piece of the puzzle. How I present myself with grace, compassion, kindness, and fun is the other big part that has happened as a result of my transformation through the *Three to Be™ Program*. My food allergy card has helped me set myself free from the shame around my allergies because it has helped me speak my truth.

Feel free to reach out to me at SoniaHunt.com if you want to explore making your own customized card. I'd love to help you!

So, where do we go from here? From the moment I set out on this journey and throughout the process of creating the *Three to Be*™ *Program*, I knew that all of this work had a higher purpose. That purpose was to educate others about food allergies and to prevent anyone else from suffering as I have for most of my life. In the next and final step of being safe, I come back to my roots and what life is all about: love, human connection, and being there to help each other. It's our ability to celebrate our differences that connects us as humans. My journey to achieving my North Star took on a new form of being safe through outreach, advocacy, and empathy...all in the cause of humanizing food allergies.

Stories of Wisdom on Humanizing Food Allergies

What does it mean to humanize food allergies and what advice do you have on how we can do this?

Dr. Kari Nadeau, M.D., Ph.D., FAAAAI

"Studying food allergies is more than understanding immune responses under a microscope—it involves understanding the social and emotional experiences of the food-allergic individual as well as the people who care for them. Food is a cultural, social, and physiological necessity in our world, so it follows that the significant apprehension caused by food allergies must be addressed during the pursuit of new treatments and investigations into the causes of food allergies.

Understanding the three-dimensional aspects of food allergies requires partnership, communication, and collaboration across fields and disciplines. The academic research community must work with the pharmaceutical and food industries, who all in turn must center on the experiences of patients themselves.

We are making strides across a wide array of therapeutics, from allergen immunotherapies to vaccines and anti-IgE drugs. Considering the impact of these interventions on patients provides important context for my work. In my own clinical research center, patients and families work with psychologists and a diverse team of clinicians and researchers who provide patient-centered care tailored to the needs of each unique family.

The prevalence of food allergies is a marker of racial and socioeconomic disparities as well, with higher rates of asthma and allergy in Black individuals in the United States. Food insecurity can also exacerbate the difficulty of managing a food allergy. One of my goals is to provide solutions on a population level to target specific groups who face systemic adversity.

I am focused on helping to usher in a 'new era' in the world of food allergies, which cannot be accomplished via scientific advances alone. Patients and communities provide essential insight into the personal experience of living with a food allergy. Together, I am hopeful that we can continue to integrate the human and scientific aspects of food allergies to achieve multifaceted and comprehensive solutions."

TWELVE

Humanizing Food Allergies

"... all big changes in human history have been arrived at slowly and through many compromises."

— ELEANOR ROOSEVELT

LEARNINGS

In this chapter, we'll explore that yes, it *does* take a village and that we all can learn from each other when it comes to topics that affect us personally. You'll learn:

- Humanizing food allergies is a movement.

- Divergent worldviews and lenses allow us to approach food allergy issues in slightly different and entirely positive ways.

- By humanizing food allergies, you can collect a wealth of data that will allow you to improve how you manage your allergies.

MY EARLY YEARS

During the year I spent with hives, my close friends became as sick of the hives as I did. That was because I refused to go out and let anyone see me in my hideous state. Typically, one of my besties and I played the role of wranglers, getting the crew together for Friday nights out eating, dancing, and whatnot. But with me sitting at home and not partaking, well, the party just wasn't as fun. Or at least that's what I was told when my bestie called me one day and ranted about how annoyed she was that I wasn't coming out to have fun and meet guys.

"Who the hell would want to date Jabba the Hutt?" I asked.

"Anyone would be so lucky! But you won't know unless you came out," she replied.

The thought of being at a bar—albeit with my close friends *but* also where other people could see me—was not appealing, nor was it going to happen. During those same weeks that my bestie was trying to convince me to go out, I began to see a pattern with my medications: there was a window between seven and ten o'clock p.m. when my hives would reduce a bit before coming back in a rage. In speaking with my doctors, it seemed that the medication timing was such that the meds were doing their job to suppress my hives, but then right before the next big dose, they would flare up again.

I made the mistake of telling my bestie about this.

"Perfect! So, that means you're like Cinderella—you can be at the bar drinking a martini at seven and be home by ten!" she said.

I had to admit that her train of thought wasn't wrong.

She proceeded to tell me that we'd make a pact: she'd leave with me so that I could be home by ten o'clock to take my next dose.

"Well, but what if a hive decides to appear at 9:37 p.m. and I'm talking to a guy?" I asked.

"I'll keep an eye on you, and if I see it, I'll give you a hand motion to ABORT!" she replied. "Just remember Soni, hives are the accessory of '09. Wear them loud and proud for all to see!"

How could I argue with that? Especially when someone loves you so much that they would go through everything with you. The "loud and proud" concept was interesting at the time, because I wanted to be out there but still was not. However, at the insistence of lovely humans such as my bestie, I slowly did begin to show my face—even with the hives all over it—and answer the multitude of questions about what was wrong with me. Seeing it in the moment but hearing me speak about how it was "no big deal" changed the conversation.

Fast-forward to after the hives had completely left me. I was anxious and excited about going out, beginning with dining! Now that I had a new way of doing things and a cool food allergy card ready to go, I contacted the usual suspects: the group of friends who were with me in 2008 at that Last Supper dinner. I invited them over to my house for a home-cooked dinner party and a show-and-tell exercise I was hoping they would find to be fun.

I wanted to show off my new food allergy card and talk them through how I was looking forward to "being out there" again and tell them that with their help, I was going to once again partake in fun things like dining out and going to parties. I wasn't sure these friends had ever seen an EpiPen®—let alone if they knew how to administer one if needed—so that was part of the evening's agenda as well. During apps and cocktails, I brought everyone up to speed on the current state of my allergies and the journey I was now on. I showed them my food allergy card and my EpiPen®. "My EpiPen® is always in my purse," I said, "and I'm officially giving you permission to grab it if needed and help me. And tonight, we're gonna do some role-playing." My announcement of the role-playing caused excitement (probably in the wrong sense), but this was a jokester group of friends. "Who knows what an EpiPen® is and where it goes?" I asked.

"It's a super long needle that goes into your heart. I saw it in *Pulp Fiction*, Soni. Don't worry, I got you!" a friend proclaimed. Damn, it was gonna be a long night.

I proceeded to tell my silly friend that an EpiPen® doesn't get shoved into the heart—rather it gets injected into the mid to upper leg, at a right angle perpendicular to the thigh. "Through your jeans? 'Cause you know, we can have your jeans off lickety-split if need be," another male friend chimed in.

We all laughed. Who said this process had to be boring? After the jokes, I proceeded in all seriousness with the instructions and ended by saying, "So, if I am in anaphylaxis or telling you I need help, do *not* hesitate to inject me!"

We all took turns using the Test Auto-Injector (it comes in the EpiPen® box) on my thigh, to make sure each person knew what they were doing. We even role-played the opposite way where I administered the Test Auto-Injector on their thighs. There were many questions, but we had a blast and I felt comfortable that everyone was on the same playing field now.

For weeks thereafter, a random friend would ask to try again to make sure they were getting it right and were prepared for any situation that could arise when dining with me. I revisited my instructions every two years and also when I changed to the Auvi-Q® Injector, which was smaller and more user-friendly. In the years to come, this group went above and beyond without my asking. They made sure that their own dinner parties, kids' birthday parties, and—here's the real kicker—even a wedding were *all* free of items that I was allergic to! Now, if that isn't love from your support team, I don't know what is.

If they were hosting a dinner at a restaurant, they would ask for a copy of my latest food allergy card and send it to the restaurant ahead of time, making sure I was taken care of. Once, a friend even said, "That server gave me a bad vibe! I think we should leave and go somewhere else" when we were at a restaurant. They were so proud that I had come such a long way. A ride or die crew will always watch over each other and take care of each other, prepared to deal with anything that life throws at any member of the crew—and they'll always do it with some humor.

Over the last ten years, each member of my support team has gone through their own health issues. Some developed food sensitivities, intolerances, and even allergies! Who woulda thunk it? They've come to me for advice about allergy testing and asked questions about my transformation process and how to create one for themselves. My answer was "Wait for my book!"

CHANGING INTENTIONS ON ADVOCACY AFTER 2008

In its truest sense, advocating for my food allergies was about me becoming empowered and speaking up for my health. But through this process, I discovered another intention: I wanted to use my empowerment to teach the world about food allergies and how they can be overcome using microsteps that can heal our physical, mental, spiritual, and emotional well-being. This was about driving change for humanity and stopping the food in America from making us sick and even killing us. And this movement is not something that's only associated with me, a sufferer of severe food allergies—this can be a movement for each and every one of us.

In creating my *Three to Be™ Program*, I have met thousands of people around the world who are struggling with food-related health issues. These people are looking for answers, inspiration, and actual steps on how they can *Be Healthy, Be Safe + Be Well™*. Therefore, my intention to humanize food allergies has meant that I would step up and serve as a guide to others in their journey by lending them the knowledge, support, and expertise I had gained throughout the process of working on my own well-being. It was now my turn to give back!

HOW I HUMANIZED FOOD ALLERGIES

Over the past ten years, I have spent every moment I've had outside of work meeting people and having conversations around food allergies to drive awareness and change. This included running around to restaurants and food and wine festivals and having meetings with food and entertainment magazine publishers in an effort to share my story and get their viewpoints on change. If you think back to 2010, even the concept of gluten-free foods wasn't yet a big notion in mainstream media! My intention was to try to get media professionals who didn't cover food allergies to give it some thought and airtime. During that decade, I also began blogging on my personal website about the restaurants that would help me. I even took pictures of waitstaff holding up my allergy card and posted those pics on social media to show them some love.

With perseverance, my story made it through the ranks of *Food & Wine* magazine and onto the then-current editor's desk, as I had hopes that magazines such as this could begin covering the food allergy angle for its readers. At the time, the celebrity chef culture was on the rise, yet there weren't any shows on *The Food Network*, *The Cooking Channel* or other mainstream food television that showcased cooking with food allergies. I was pitching different media companies the idea that there should be. Intrigued by my story, I became a guest chef in a series collaboration between *Food & Wine* magazine and Holland America Cruise lines. Ecstatic at the opportunity, I created an interactive demonstration called "Spicy Slim™" that taught the cruising guests how to cook healthy ethnic foods using substitutions whenever food restrictions called for them. The demo was a hit on the cruise and a great data point for this type of content, as many audience members shared their dietary restrictions and appreciation for tips on substitutions. Thereafter, I began teaching the "Spicy Slim™" class one-on-one to people struggling with food restrictions and cooking. Teaching those classes also allowed me to connect with others and share my story.

One of the biggest wins that came out of my work to humanize food allergies was my creation of "Food Allergy Dinners." These were private dinners held around the United States in partnership with a celebrity chef of my choosing. The idea was that the chef and I would partner up to present a conversation about what restaurants can do to handle food allergies and how to share information between the diner and the restaurant before, during, and after the experience. I chose chefs who also had a personal story related to food restrictions and supported what I was trying to do. There was time to mingle as guests arrived, and during cocktails, I built in time to discuss topics laid out on the table about food and health during the ensuing allergen-friendly dinner. These events allowed people with diverse backgrounds to come together and have discussions about a topic that was interesting to them: food restrictions and health.

I was so proud of this partnership with chefs! I also promoted them and their restaurants because of all they had done to help me. The very first dinner was co-hosted with Chef Alexander Ong at Betelnut Restaurant in San Francisco. He featured a delectable and allergy-friendly Singaporean-style dinner. Other dinners were in partnership with the James Beard-winning Vetri Team in my hometown of Philadelphia, including Chefs Brad Spence and Jeff Michaud at Amis Trattoria, and also with the always-vibrant Chef Fabio Viviani of Top Chef Fame in Los Angeles, in addition to others. These lovely people became friends and helped me spread the news and the love by helping others like me who came to dine in their restaurants. I will forever be grateful to them.

The dinners were promoted on social media and through email lists, and I donated all of the proceeds to food allergy research. Interestingly and according to my data, most who attended these dinners did not have diagnosed food allergies but were interested in the topic and how restaurants handled restrictions. It was awesome to know that I was hitting a new target audience!

> **THE CULMINATION OF MUCH WORK CAME IN 2015, WHEN I WAS ASKED TO SPEAK ON THE TEDX PLATFORM ABOUT MY PERSONAL STORY. DREAMS REALLY DO COME TRUE!**

HOW YOU CAN HUMANIZE FOOD ALLERGIES

I need you to know that *any* form of advocacy or humanization of food allergies will never be seen as small. This is your personal journey and not a competition with others, so do what you feel you can. I was on a personal mission, and you can be, too. My recommendation is to dream big and use your journal or whiteboard to strategize what you would like to do to drive change for others in the world of food allergies. In regard to execution, think of small things that go a long way. Here are four ways you can start:

Step One: Create Small Steps to Drive Big Impact. Take some time to determine and write down ways in which you can drive impact for the food allergy movement. Remember, you are the example for excellence in this transformation! Go into the world and show others how to do it. Could you create a yearly allergy-friendly bake sale at your school or workplace? Could you create a fun badge to hand out to restaurants in your neighborhood who are doing a great job accommodating food allergies? The idea would be that they place that badge in their window. Making an impact can be everything from speaking publicly or starting your own website/podcast to creating an app for food allergies or helping people one-on-one (my favorite!) with their daily struggles. Creating a local "March for Food Allergies" event or teaching allergy-friendly cooking classes are more great ways to begin to humanize food allergies. Remember, nothing you may decide to do is small.

Step Two: Create a "Dining In" Plan. When you are hosting a dinner party, turn the tables around by asking if anyone has any dietary restrictions ahead of time so that you can plan for it. (If you can believe it, I never used to do this because I was always the problem child.) Putting others first—especially in your own home—goes a long way toward building solid relationships and adding folks to your support team. I recommend keeping notes of the friends who have food allergies, restrictions, or dietary preferences in your journal or a spreadsheet. For those that do have restrictions, incorporate their help if you're cooking or ordering in. It's always more fun to strategize a menu with others! When you take the lead to make sure they are taken care of during a dining experience, you'll see all your hard work come to fruition firsthand.

Step Three: Create a "Dining Out" Plan. Similarly, create steps for dining out, including what you will do before, at check-in, during, and after your experience. In a restaurant situation, I recommend calling ahead of time to find out if they can accommodate you. If they can, email them a copy of your food allergy card. Once you arrive, talk to the host and remind them that you are the one with the food allergies and make a personal connection with them. Who doesn't love walking into a restaurant where they know your name! At the table, use your unique style and walk your server through your cool new food allergy card, educating them and allowing them time to think and ask questions. Then, when your food comes out to your table, I recommend reconfirming that it is void of the allergens listed on your card. Always be grateful that the staff is willing to help. Go the extra step and thank the team in the kitchen or send the restaurant an email afterward about your experience—whether good or bad and with suggestions on what needs improvement. I also highly recommend going online to offer a great review of restaurants that can accommodate allergen-free dining on tools such as Google reviews, Yelp.com, Opentable.com, and AllergyEats.com. Be open to working with them! Collaborating will go a long way toward helping you achieve what you want, which is to be safe and have a lovely dining experience.

THE NET NET

Having a sense of community unites us and makes us feel like we are part of something greater than ourselves. It can give us opportunities to connect with people and to reach for our goals, and it makes us feel safe and secure. No one person has all the answers, and when it comes to food allergies, it's not just about gaining wisdom from those who are suffering, it's also about gaining wisdom from those who don't have allergies, because diverse thoughts and opinions are needed in the fight for a cure. Through diversity, we grow, and our divergent worldviews and lenses mean that each of us approaches the exact same problem slightly differently.

When we work alone, it's often easy to give up on things when the going gets tough. But when you surround yourself with others working toward a similar goal or objective, you'll get motivation, support, and friendly competition that will cause you to push yourself just a *bit* further than you would have on your own. And on those days when you just want to give up, leaning into your community and support team will show you how amazing you are and that you got this!

So, where do we go from here? As they say in *Looney Tunes*, "That's all, folks!" Just kidding. Come on, aren't you a wee bit interested in how creating and utilizing my *Three to Be™ Program* turned out for me? Then I'll see ya in the final chapter for all the juicy details!

But before we get there, let's look back to the 3x3 matrix of the *Three to Be™ Program* that were covered in chapters 4-12. To recap, this program has three main principles of *Healthy, Safe + Well,* and three steps within each principle.

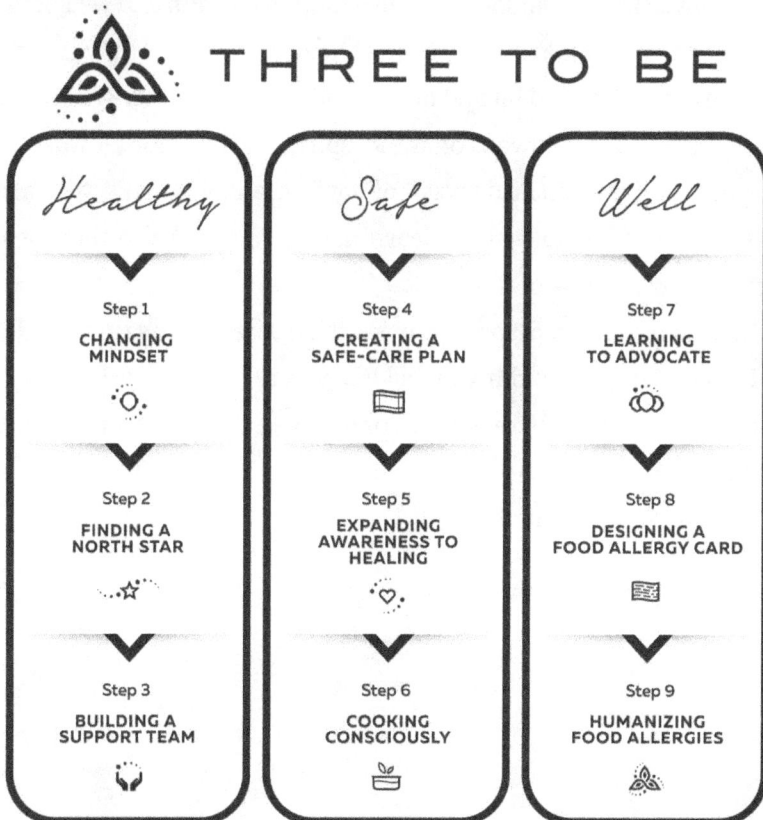

THREE TO BE

Healthy	*Safe*	*Well*
Step 1 CHANGING MINDSET	**Step 4** CREATING A SAFE-CARE PLAN	**Step 7** LEARNING TO ADVOCATE
Step 2 FINDING A NORTH STAR	**Step 5** EXPANDING AWARENESS TO HEALING	**Step 8** DESIGNING A FOOD ALLERGY CARD
Step 3 BUILDING A SUPPORT TEAM	**Step 6** COOKING CONSCIOUSLY	**Step 9** HUMANIZING FOOD ALLERGIES

Think of the principles as life themes, whereas each step within a principle is how you accomplish that theme. For example, in order to be healthy, you'll be taking steps to change mindset, find a North Star, and build a support team—and so on. The intention of this program is to *Be Free*—free from trauma, free from health issues, free from food allergies, free to be me (as I like to say). I took the time to create, try, test and tweak each of these steps for years until it was working like a machine. Just as life happens, I evolved along with the evolution of this program. Yes, it takes time, but in the process, I learned so many wonderful things about myself, and with daily microsteps in each of these areas, I viscerally felt myself flourish.

The *Three to Be™ Program* is about reclaiming your life holistically. Its core is centered around a desire to *Be Healthy, Be Safe + Be Well™* across physical, mental, spiritual, and emotional health and well-being. After focusing primarily on physical health for most of my life, the other areas took a hard hit and held me back from healing. By allowing myself to also focus inward on mind, spirit, and emotions, I was able to heal, break free, and rid myself of my food allergies. This work also then allowed me to take all my learnings outward to help others heal, which is the purpose of this book.

You can begin at Step 1 and work the entire process through just as I did or jump around if you feel like you're already working some of the steps. Again, there is no wrong way to do you! Your personal well-being is just that—it's personal to you.

Onwards, to the final chapter!

PART V

Final Words

THIRTEEN

Free to Be Me

"Freeing yourself was one thing; claiming ownership
of that freed self was another."

—TONI MORRISON

Transformation takes time, patience, heart, and hell of a lot
of gusto. It is much easier to repeat rather than evolve. But I
wouldn't have been me if I hadn't said I was going to do this and then
make good on my promise to the Universe! I began creating the *Three
to Be™ Program* after my 2008 incident, and once I had the foundation, I
jumped in and worked it, testing and tweaking it as I learned. Over the
course of ten years, I kept trying to hit my North Star. As we approached
the end of the 2010s, I wanted to go in peace and welcome what was
to come in a new decade. I decided to do that in meditation, reflecting
on how I have persevered.

In December 2019, I sat for my very first Vipassana, which is one
of India's most ancient techniques of meditation and one that focuses
on the deep interconnection between mind and body. Vipassana[80] has
been taught in India for more than 2,500 years as a universal remedy
for universal ills. The 12-day program I sat for consisted of:

- A vow of noble silence

- No contact with other humans

- No devices whatsoever

- No journals or reading materials

- Four o' clock a.m. wake-up calls

- Two vegetarian meals per day

- 14 hours of Vipassana meditation practice per day

I know what you're saying—"This girl truly is a nut job! Why in the world would anyone want to do that?" Well, I thought the same thing for many years. I won't lie: Vipassana is incredibly difficult and not for the faint of heart. But I was looking to round out a period of incredible growth with some alone time to soak it all in and be proud of everything I had accomplished.

> **WITH A CHANGED MINDSET, I WENT FROM TELLING THE UNIVERSE WHAT I WANTED FROM IT, TO ASKING THE UNIVERSE WHAT IT WANTED FROM ME.**

According to the Vipassana Research Institute, "Vipassana enables us to experience peace and harmony by purifying the mind, freeing it from suffering and the deep-seated causes of suffering. Step by step, the practice leads to the highest spiritual goal of full liberation from all mental defilements".[81] I had just gone through a renewal of body, mind, spirit, and emotions in creating the *Three to Be™ Program*, and I was on a path to enlightenment.

Ironically, as I headed home from my Vipassana experience, COVID-19 was just hitting the world. Little did I know that we'd all be entering a year of isolation, a year when my physical, mental, spiritual, and emotional well-being would be put to its greatest test yet. For the first time in my life, I was ready, prepared, and in control of my own destiny. *Nothing* was going to take me back to negative ways, not even a little biatch named COVID-19.

In my past life, I have felt as small and insignificant as humanly possible, hurting and aching in places I didn't even know I had inside me. But I overcame all of it; I realized a new purpose in life and I was able to thrive even in the madness of 2020. I could do that because great health is a case of mind over matter.

EVOLUTION OF AN INDIAN-AMERICAN FAMILY

My parents adapted in order to raise a child with severe food allergies and asthma, and then evolved alongside me once when I started my new journey. For sure they thought I was a bit nutty for putting myself through such a rigorous process here, one that was grueling and at times manifested in me hysterically calling them, upset when things were difficult. They accepted their new role of being partners in my process and trusted that I knew what I was doing—after all, they had taught me well. As partners, they listened, learned, and heard me in a new way, which allowed them to advise me appropriately when I asked them to. As a result, they were able to witness their child owning her situation, becoming empowered, speaking her truth, and maneuvering through life in a careful, thoughtful, and joyous way. This process was totally different from our Indian culture's definition of a parent-child relationship where the parent says and the child does, no questions asked. I commend them for being willing and able to become my partners in this process.

As a partnership is a two-way relationship, in return, I became their personal concierge to all things related to food and health, expanding their minds. I became an Encyclopedia Brown of everything gluten-free so that I could help family members dealing with gluten issues. I did the research, talked to the experts, tested every possible gluten-free product I could find, and documented my findings so that I could share the information. My dad and I had always bonded over diet and exercise and how he could utilize alternative ingredients in his own food plan to ward off future ailments. When I found healthy alternative products, I would test them out in my own cooking and then send home a box of those products for my parents to try.

My transformation pushed my parents to grow in many ways, and together, we blended the best parts of East meets West in each of our holistic healing plans.

TO 10 THINGS I CULTIVATED OVER MY TRANSFORMATION

Using the *Three to Be™ Program* for holistic healing added value to every single aspect of my life. I could fill another book with all of my learnings! Here are my Top 10:

1. Being broken is a choice.
2. Life with food allergies is about more than just the food we put into our bodies—it is about our body, mind, spirit, and emotions aligning together to live with intent and purpose.
3. All humans have the right to eat food that neither makes us sick nor kills us.
4. Understanding our truths and finding the courage to speak them is at the core of transformation.
5. Everybody brings something of value to the table, and we are not here to judge that value.
6. Conscious decision-making is imperative for our health and well-being.

7. When we understand that our behaviors, patterns, and habits are a result of unconscious programming, only then can we deconstruct where they came from in order to free ourselves.

8. Letting go of expectations is fundamental to living an unencumbered life.

9. Surrounding yourself with legendary souls who inspire you to dive deeper, love harder, express bravery, and show up more sparkly will help you open your soul to the world.

10. Every moment is a learning opportunity. Remain teachable.

THE NET NET...HOW ARE MY FOOD ALLERGIES TODAY?

The year 2021 marked 13 years after my 2008 incident. I started the year full of life and with a tingling feeling all over. But this time that tingling was a great one. January 21, 2021 was an auspicious day: A friend told me that at exactly 9:21pm that day, it was the 21st minute of the 21st hour of the 21st day of the 21st year of the 21st century! That had to mean something good.

But the main event on January 21 was this: after three rounds of testing many months apart which began during the previous year, I was told by my doctors that my food allergies were gone. *All of them.* They were eliminated, or, as my allergist put it, "They are in remission." #BYEFELICIA!

With eyes wide open and in complete and utter shock, all that came out of my mouth was, "Say what?"

We first received these results in 2020, but I didn't believe them. So, I had two different doctors run them twice, months apart. Both sets of results came back the same, but I still wasn't convinced. Talk about a Nut Job! Since 2021 was the 13th year after my 2008 incident, I asked my doctors to run full skin and IgE blood testing yet again to validate for a final time. And for a third time the results concluded that it truly was my Lucky 13!

Peanuts: gone. Tree nuts: gone. Avocado, banana, halibut: gone, gone, gone! And so on. Every single one of my food allergies either ranged from undetectable to low level at the highest which is why my allergist said it seems they are now in remission.

Furthermore, we also ran IgE allergen component blood testing on any of my allergic foods where component testing was available (including peanuts, walnuts, and hazelnuts), which looks at the offending allergens on the molecular level. These tests tell doctors which individual proteins of a particular food, such as peanuts, for example, the patient is sensitized to. There are eight levels to this form of testing, with the lowest being "Absent/Undetectable" and the highest being "Very High Level." My peanuts and tree nuts results were "Absent/Undetectable," and some other foods like banana and avocado were "Very Low Level." Thus, in reviewing all of the test results, the consensus from my doctors was that my food allergies were now gone. Food Allergy Research & Education reports that, "Allergies to peanuts, tree nuts, fish and shellfish are generally lifelong".[82]

I have officially beat the odds.

SKIN TEST RESULTS

www.theallergyclinic.com

Name: Sonia Hunt   DOB: _____   Date: 1·21·21

FOOD TESTING

A			B			C			D		
1	Almond	2	1	Bean, Navy	1-2	1	Cantaloupe	(-)	1	Cinnamon	(-)
2	Apricot	(-)	2	Bean, String	(-)	2	Carrot		2	Clam	
3	Apple		3	Beef		3	Casein		3	Coconut	
4	Asparagus		4	Black Bass		4	Cashew		4	Codfish	
5	Histamine	4	5	Black Pepper		5	Catfish		5	Coffee	
6	Saline	(-)	6	Blueberry		6	Cauliflower		6	Corn	
7	Avocado		7	Brazil Nut		7	Celery		7	Crab	
8	Banana		8	Broccoli		8	Cherry		8	Cranberry	
9	Barley		9	Buckwheat		9	Chicken Meat		9	Cucumber	
10	Lima Bean	1	10	Cabbage		10	Chocolate		10	Egg, White	

E			F			G			H		
1	Egg, Yolk	(-)	1	Hazelnut	1	1	Milk, Goat	(-)	1	Pear	(-)
2	Flounder		2	Honeydew	(-)	2	Mushroom		2	Pecan Nut	
3	Garlic		3	Hops		3	Mustard		3	Perch	
4	Ginger		4	Lamb		4	Nutmeg		4	Pineapple	
5	Grape, White		5	Lemon		5	Oat, Grain		5	Pistachio Nut	
6	Grapefruit		6	Lettuce		6	Onion		6	Plum	
7	Green Olive		7	Lobster		7	Orange		7	Pork	
8	Green Pea		8	Mackerel		8	Oyster		8	Potato, Sweet	
9	Green Bell Pepper		9	Malt		9	Peach		9	Potato, White	
10	Halibut		10	Milk, Cow		10	Peanut		10	Rice	

I			J		
1	Raspberry	(-)	1	Tea	(-)
2	Rye, Grain		2	Tomato	
3	Salmon		3	Trout	
4	Scallop		4	Tuna	
5	Sesame		5	Turkey	
6	Shrimp		6	Vanilla	
7	Soybean		7	Walnut, English	
8	Spinach		8	Watermelon	
9	Squash		9	Wheat, Grain	
10	Strawberry		10	Yeast	

Pertinent Positives:

- Ø See Select Foods   O Nuts
- O Fruits/Vegetables   O Seafood
- O Meats   O Grains

Number of Allergen Units Tested: 100

Performed by: _____

Read by: _____

MD Signature: _____

Form Revised: 12/29/17

COMPONENT TESTING LEGEND

Endnote 1

Specific IGE Class	kU/L	Level of Allergen Specific IGE Antibody
0	<0.10	Absent/Undetectable
0/1	0.10-0.34	Very Low Level
1	0.35-0.69	Low Level
2	0.70-3.49	Moderate Level
3	3.50-17.4	High Level
4	17.5-49.9	Very High Level
5	50-100	Very High Level
6	>100	Very High Level

The clinical relevance of allergen results of 0.10-0.34 kU/L are undetermined and intended for specialist use.

Allergens denoted with a "**" include results using one or more analyte specific reagents. In those cases, the test was developed and its analytical performance characteristics have been determined by Quest Diagnostics. It has not been cleared or approved by the U.S. Food and Drug Administration. This assay has been validated pursuant to the CLIA regulations and is used for clinical purposes.

COMPONENT TESTING RESULTS

Quest Diagnostics	Page	01/29/2021 12:49:36 PM	**Report Status: Final - Courtesy Copy**
			HUNT, SONIA

Patient Information	Specimen Information	Client Information
HUNT, SONIA	Specimen:	Client #:
	Collected: 01/22/2021 / 11:08 PST	
DOB: **AGE:**	Received: 01/23/2021 / 03:21 PST	
Gender: F Fasting: Y	Faxed: 01/29/2021 / 12:46 PST	
Patient ID:		
Health ID:		

WALNUT COMPONENT PANEL
Lab: UL

Test Name	Results	Reference Range
rJug r1 (f441)	<0.10	<0.10 kU/L
rJug r3 (f442)	<0.10	<0.10 kU/L

IgE reactivity to whole walnut without reactivity to the Jug r 1 or Jug r 3 may be explained by IgE reactivity to other walnut proteins, cross-reactive pollen proteins, or cross-reactive carbohydrates.

HAZELNUT COMPONENT PANEL
Lab: UL

Test Name	Results	Reference Range
Cor a1 (f428)	<0.10	<0.10 kU/L
Cor a8 (f425)	<0.10	<0.10 kU/L
Cor a9 (f440)	<0.10	<0.10 kU/L
Cor a14 (f439)	<0.10	<0.10 kU/L

IgE reactivity to whole hazelnut without reactivity to the hazelnut component(s) tested may be explained by IgE reactivity to other hazelnut proteins, cross-reactive pollen proteins, or cross-reactive carbohydrates.

PEANUT COMPONENT PANEL
Lab: UL

Test Name	Results	Reference Range
Ara h 2 (f423)	<0.10	<0.10 kU/L
Ara h 1 (f422)	<0.10	<0.10 kU/L
Ara h 3 (f424)	<0.10	<0.10 kU/L
Ara h 9 (f427)	<0.10	<0.10 kU/L
Ara h 8 (f352)	<0.10	<0.10 kU/L

Reactivity to whole peanut without reactivity to the peanut component(s) tested may be explained by IgE reactivity to other peanut proteins, cross-reactive pollen proteins, or cross-reactive carbohydrates.

PERFORMING SITE:
UL   QUEST DIAGNOSTICS SACRAMENTO, 3714 NORTHGATE BLVD, SACRAMENTO, CA 95834-1617 Laboratory Director: M ROSE AKIN, M.D., FCAP, CLIA: 05D0644206

I, Sonia Hunt, ecstatically proclaim that I have hit my North Star and have healthily eliminated ALL of my food allergies!!! Wheeeee! I know you are dancing in celebratory spirit with me! Additionally, I am tickled pink to report that I have not had an emergency room visit since 2008 and that my asthma has gone into a dormant state as well. My deep focus and hard work made it happen, and I am overjoyed to share this news with you!

The *Three to Be™ Program* was a complete deconstruction and reconstruction of me. A five-ingredient recipe led to this moment:

Ingredient One: Will. I created the conditions to heal myself, plain and simple. And you can, too.

Ingredient Two: A Focus on Holistic Health. Making a change to focus on my body, mind, spirit, and emotions together completely changed my life. I always knew that healing was about more than just abstaining from foods—I hypothesized that if I could heal other areas affecting my allergies, then I could heal my food allergies as well. The years of detailed research and testing with doctors about my situation netted out at this conclusion: at the root of my food allergies were genetic predispositions, environmental factors, and intestinal permeabilities. This information allowed me to try various herbal remedies and whole-body practices from Ayurvedic and functional medicine that specifically worked to heal and strengthen at the root level. This allowed me to get off Western medications for the long run, which was very important to me.

Ingredient Three: Diet and Exercise. Making deep, conscious changes to my diet on the ingredient and source levels truly allowed me to heal. I relearned how to cook and eat holistically. Understanding that certain types of diets also benefited the planet was freeing. Using new and different forms of movement to work on my overall health and improve my gut health and asthma was also key.

Ingredient Four: Outgrowing Food Allergies Over Time.
I always prayed this would happen, but it was a long while in the making. During the years leading up to 2008, my testing showed that my food allergies remained severe even though I was not having active reactions often. From 2008 onwards, they continued to show up as very severe in my testing. It was only in the last few years (~2017 onwards) that my test results showed reduced levels of varying allergies—so we concluded that the changed management of my food allergies seemed to be working. Remember, I was the unusual case: someone who got more and more food allergies as I aged. But by focusing on holistic health through diet and exercise, my body finally began to heal itself from years of toxicity.

Ingredient Five: A Little Luck. Yes, I believe that luck flows around in the Universe like a beautiful breeze, but I worked really really hard to make that luck ticket finally arrive.

After four decades of living with severe food allergies, a new journey has started! This journey is rooted in all things that allow me to be healthy, safe, and well. When COVID-19 hit the world in 2020, even with my positive results I purposely stayed extra-precautious and chose to keep my Auvi-Q Injector®, Benadryl®, and a steroid inhaler on hand for emergency purposes. But *not* having to use them during perhaps the scariest year in my lifetime was incredibly freeing.

Years ago, I had identified my North Star: *To age healthily by ridding myself of my food allergies.* So, have I accomplished this? You bet your ass I have! And no, this does not mean that I'm going to start having plates of peanut butter and jelly sandwiches or that I'm going to sit in a corner snacking on SNICKERS® bars or M&M'S® Peanut Chocolate Candy. For the rest of my life, I will stay conscious about what goes into and onto my body. But now I can breathe a sigh of relief and begin to figure out what life looks like for me going forward. I will still ask questions about what's in a dish and I will still read labels because I am health-conscious.

I will take this process slowly; one day soon, I'll choose whether or not to safely incorporate the foods I was once allergic to into my life. Participating in food challenges with my allergist is one avenue I can go down if I feel the need to eat nuts. But to be honest, I don't even remember what a peanut tastes like and I may just not want to go there. This is about progress and a big celebration soon to come!

Could my allergies come back again one day? It's anyone's guess. But over the past decade leading up to my 2021 diagnosis of freedom, I saw signs that my allergies had been reducing. My future will always include continuing to work my *Three to Be™ Program* to age healthily knowing that I have other genetic predispositions to consider. None of those are in my life yet, but they should watch out, 'cause I'm coming for them if they do appear!

So, where do we go from here? There is a mindfulness component to having food allergies, as you have to be in the moment and aware before you put something into your mouth. That can be debilitating even for the strong-minded, but if you flip the script, it can lead you towards a path of enlightenment. It's important to note that joy did not happen to me only at the end, when I found out that my allergies were gone. Joy has happened all throughout this process, because I have completely transformed. People always ask me, "How do you look so young?" I say it's because I have invested time into healing, loving myself, and making myself better so that I can be better for the world. I healed the inside, and that inner healing has manifested into me being a vibrant human on the outside. And *that*, my friends, is the true fountain of youth.

One additional thing I will say is that although we were all rocked to our core during COVID-19, the pandemic changed something incredibly important: restaurants operated at their highest levels of cleanliness and sanitation to accommodate everyone. Now all of us know firsthand what it means for restaurants to operate at a level where they must keep themselves—*all* of their employees and *all* of their customers—safe from harm. This is HUGE news for the food allergy community. We always knew this could happen!

WE MUST CONTINUE TO PUSH FORWARD THIS SAME LEVEL OF SERVICE FOR PEOPLE DINING WITH FOOD ALLERGIES.

The word "serendipity," or a series of fortunate accidents, is one of my all-time fave words. In my case, serendipity was the Last Supper dinner in 2008, which started a tsunami of events that took me from almost dying to making a life transformation. Sometimes the scars we can't see are the ones that hurt the most. I no longer wanted to live with those scars nor worry about what was or wasn't going to happen, so I worked hard toward achieving balance in all areas of my life. All of the testing, hives, hospital visits, pain, trauma, and shame that I went through for years were absolutely amazing teachers that helped me transform and know that my best was yet to come.

The Riverside Church of New York City published a sermon by Minister Ernest T. Campbell delivered on January 25, 1970. An excerpt from that sermon was later published in the novel *Boulder Reveries* by W. S. Blatchley. Blatchley quotes Minister Campbell as saying, "Our times call not for diction but for action. It has been said that the two most important days of a man's life are the day on which he was born and the day on which he discovers why he was born. This is why we were born: To love the Lord our God with all our heart and soul and mind and strength, and our neighbor as ourselves".[83] Throughout my transformation, I realized that I am on this Earth to bring light and love to other beings. I am not a medical professional, but I have deep experience managing food allergies, environmental allergies and asthma for four decades. The information in this book is what worked for me. I share this information with you so that I can support you through your health challenges, by taking small steps and receiving big love along the way. All of this allows me to be the greatest version of Sonia Hunt that the world has ever seen.

Applying the steps of my *Three to Be™ Program* can not only greatly improve your holistic health but also your life. So, I challenge you to open your mind and work the program! There is no wrong way to work the program, and only you get to choose how to go about it. Just be curious and do everything with full consciousness.

I wish that you have the kind of results I have received. But regardless of your results, I wish you are able to transform in a way to live each day healthily and joyously. Always know that I'm with you should you need a cheerleader, a ridiculously smiley friend, or a coach—just reach out to me at SoniaHunt.com. I got you.

Resources

CREATE AN INSTANT FOOD ALLERGY CARD

If you don't yet have a food allergy card, I got ya covered! Here are two pop-out templates for an instant food allergy card. Just fill in your information, cut around the edges and begin to use it every time you're dining. I recommend taking this to your local printer to laminate it so it's easy to clean off spilled food.

Name_____   **FOOD ALLERGY CARD**

Foods	Flours & Oils	Medications
_____	_____	_____
_____	_____	_____
_____	_____	_____
_____	_____	_____
_____	_____	_____
_____	_____	_____
_____	_____	_____

Caution: *I have food allergies. Please use clean gloves, utensils, surfaces and cookware when creating my meal. Thanks!*

⚜ **911** ⚜

Mom _____
Dad _____

Name_____   **FOOD ALLERGY CARD**

Foods	
Flours & Oils	
Medications	

Caution: *I have food allergies. Please use clean gloves, utensils, surfaces and cookware when creating my meal. Thanks!*

⚜ **911** ⚜

Mom _____
Dad _____

ACKNOWLEDGEMENTS

On many days, this book was the bane of my existence. Had it not been for the gorgeous souls who believed in me, understood when I declined attending their party for the tenth time, yet encouraged me to keep writing!—I wouldn't have been able to finish this book. It truly did take a village to make it happen! I am so grateful to everyone who has touched my life with food allergies, and will continue to do so.

To Kassius Marcellus Hunt, who never left my side or lap, and only minimally whined that I was on the computer 24/7 to write this book. I love you #morethanlife!

This book would not have come together if it were not for the gifted humans who like magic, shared their craft with me. To my editor, Julie Artz, for being an amazing partner and guiding me to make sense of all the stuff in my head (and for not getting annoyed when I asked a million times, "Are these commas correct?"). I am so grateful to you for helping me bring this story to life. To my copy editor, Lisa Howard, for your spectacular attention to detail, and shared interests in holistic health. To my graphic design team, Aleksandar Nikodinovski for the *Three to Be™ Program*, and Jasmine Hromjak for my interior book layout and helping me to finalize my book cover: I'm so grateful to both of you for being in the weeds with me to bring my vision to life. To Erika Heald and Maureen Jann, for your strategic minds and thoughtfulness with my brand.

To the beautiful ladies who shared their personal stories for this book: Robyn O'Brien, Emily Brown, Sarah Krahenbuhl, Dina Hawthorne-Silvera, Dr. Jill Carnahan, M.D., Colleen Kavanaugh, Riya Miglani, Eleanor Garrow-Holding, Dr. Kari Nadeau, MD, PhD.. You have led the path, and I will always be inspired by your devotion to helping others with food allergies.

To my family who has provided for a lifetime of laughter, fun stories and experiences, I love you dearly: my maternal and paternal grandparents, the Acharya family, the Arte family, the Rajpathak family, the Londhe family, the Pradhan family, the Karnik family, the Talim family, the Kamerkar family, the Keer family, my long list of cousins on both sides, and all of my fake-cousins and bonus parents in "The Gang."

To my soulmates, my #rideordie crew, those whom I refer to as "my people,"...I love each and every one of you to pieces: Mark Karam, Christine Tjon and Jay Abellana, Julie Noto, Zeena Fakoury and Rob Doeblin, Reshma Pradhan Lensing and Bradley Lensing, Robert Mayell, Alexei Levene, Anjali Thakur, Lee Ann McLoughlin, Denise Hadley Williams and John Williams, Carolyn Dismuke, Hazel and Jeremy Bordi, Noura Fakoury, Barry Bonds, Carmina Ilagan, Jennifer and Jeff Milum, Leslie Deamer, Alexander Ong, Scott Howard, Dr. Robert Brown, M.D., Keith Brownfield, Micheal Cross Trinity, Mike Siemonsma, Seema and Devan Batavia, Jeannette Boudreau, Ketan Anjaria, Richard Bernstein, Vania Cunha, Donald Burlock, Jr., Tommy Campagne, the late Cecilia Chiang, Philip Chiang, Ratika and Puneet Chopra, Doug and Jessica Chu, Kari Lincks-Coomans and Parker Coomans, Anjali and Vivek Dighe, Tommy Filippone, Ben Fileccia, Katherine and Igor Fishbeyn, William Flaiz, Rama Krishnamoorthy and Paul Fullarton, Shilpa Gadkari, Maya Goradia, Tony Guerra, Angus Huang, Arianna Huffington, Terri and James Hnatyszyn, Rajashree and Sunil Joshi, Rajul and Alpesh Kadakia, Nicholas Keeler, Gabrielle and Craig Keeler, Marni and Raj Khanna, Akriti and Amandeep Khurana, Maryam Khotani, Jenn Lim, Sam Naimi, Gina Noto, Ronda Gabb, Nidia Vodonovich, Sonia Martinez, Nevaeh Jackson, Daisy

Chhatwal and Tanvir Mangat, Ryan Macaulay, Claire Mayell, the late Mark Mastin, Robert McCorvey, Jeff Michaud, Ramon Montemayor, Scott Morris, Hosna Tavakoli and Behnam Nader, James J. Nicholas III, Mee Mee Nguyen, Ritu Raj, Alyssa Rapp and Hal Morris, Leroy Ratnayake, Jeff Roach, Henry Odiase, Kathy O'Neal, Keyur Patel, Aanal Udayi, Parneet Pal, Sunil Paul and Mera Granberg Paul, Ann Polhemus Peltz, Monika and Gustavo E. Perez, Rachel and Santo Puranama, Jack Sammons, Dorit Sasson, Veronica Sauret, Leslie Hartley-Sbrocco, Brad Patrick Spence, Jeremy Streich, Phil Shell, Bindul Turakhia, Marc Vetri, Fabio Viviani, Mike Wells, J. Randall Williams, Max Yeh, Karen Kong, Ted Allen, Evelyn Manangan, Matthieu Meynier, Sonya Yruel, Anna Salazar, and Laurel Katz.

To my Facebook, and Instagram family, you and your kindness are always in my heart.

To the countless chefs, service staff, restaurant owners around the globe who have shown me love by helping me to eat safely while having an amazing dining experience—I am grateful to all of you.

AND FINALLY, TO EVERYONE IN THE WORLD WHO SUFFERS DUE TO SEVERE FOOD ALLERGIES AND FOOD RESTRICTIONS: THERE IS HOPE... BECAUSE *YOU ARE* THAT HOPE.

MORE FROM SONIA

To connect with Sonia and see what she's up to, go to soniahunt.com, and on social media at Facebook.com/huntsonia, Instagram @soniahunt, and Twitter @soniahunt. Also, you can view Sonia's TEDx Talk on food allergies on YouTube.

NOTES

ENDNOTES

1   http://www.fortunejournals.com/articles/environmental-factors-contribute-to-the-onset-of-food-allergies.html#:~:text=Some%20possible%20roles%20the%20environment,The%20study%20looked%20at%20children.

2   Erin Nicole Benton, Department of Health, Human Performance and Recreation, Baylor University, Waco, Texas, USA, and Christie Maria Sayes, Department of Environmental Science, Baylor University, Waco, Texas, USA, Journal of Environmental Science and Public Health, http://www.fortunejournals.com/articles/environmental-factors-contribute-to-the-onset-of-food-allergies.html#:~:text=Some%20possible%20roles%20the%20environment,The%20study%20looked%20at%20children, Published 13 July, 2017.

3   Asthma and Allergy Foundation of America, https://www.aafa.org/food-as-an-asthma-trigger.aspx

4   Erin Nicole Benton, Department of Health, Human Performance and Recreation, Baylor University, Waco, Texas, USA, and Christie Maria Sayes, Department of Environmental Science, Baylor University, Waco, Texas, USA, Journal of Environmental Science and Public Health, http://www.fortunejournals.com/articles/environmental-factors-contribute-to-the-onset-of-food-allergies.html#:~:text=Some%20possible%20roles%20the%20environment,The%20study%20looked%20at%20children, Published 13 July, 2017.

5   Sara Benede, Ana Belen Blázquez, David Chiang, Leticia Tordesillas, M. Cecilia Berin, *The Rise of Food Allergy: Environmental Factors and Emerging Treatments*, https://www.ncbi.nlm.nih.gov/pmc/articles/PMC4909486/, 16 April, 2016.

6   Dr. Ruchi Gupta, M.D., MPH, *50% of People Who Think They Have a Food Allergy Actually Don't*, https://www.technologynetworks.com/applied-sciences/news/50-of-people-who-think-they-have-a-food-allergy-actually-dont-313579, 07 January, 2019

7   Food Allergy Education & Research, *Facts and Statistics*, https://www.foodallergy.org/resources/facts-and-statistics

8   Jonathan I. Silverberg, MD, PhD, MPH; Eric L. Simpson, MD, MCR; Helen G. Durkin, PhD; Rauno Joks, MD, *Prevalence of Allergic Disease in Foreign Born American Children*, JAMA Pediatrics, JAMA Pediatr. Published online April 29, 2013. doi:10.1001/jamapediatrics.2013.1319

9   U.S. Department of Justice, Civil Rights Division, *Disability Rights Section, A Guide to Disability Rights Laws*, https://www.ada.gov/cguide.htm

10 Kristen D. Jackson, M.P.H.; LaJeana D. Howie, M.P.H., C.H.E.S.; Lara J. Akinbami, M.D., *Trends in Allergic Conditions Among Children: United States, 1997–2011*, https://www.cdc.gov/nchs/products/databriefs/db121.htm, Number 121, May 2013 https://www.cdc.gov/nchs/products/databriefs/db121.htm

[11] Steven Reinberg, *New report reveals how many Americans have food allergies,* https://www.cbsnews.com/news/food-allergies-in-america-new-report-shellfish-peanut-dairy/#:~:text=Approximately%204%20percent%20of%20Americans,%2C%22%20said%20lead%20researcher%20Dr, 01 June, 2017

[12] Tim Ferriss, https://tim.blog/podcast/

[13] Rick Hanson, rickhanson.net, https://www.rickhanson.net/find-your-north-star/

[14] Goodreads.com, https://www.goodreads.com/quotes/103315-the-wound-is-the-place-where-the-light-enters-you

[15] Dictionary.com, https://www.dictionary.com/browse/survivor?s=t

[16] Alex Macpherson, The Guardian, *'I saw my life going down a drain',* https://www.theguardian.com/music/2008/feb/01/urban, *31 January, 2008,*

[17] James R. Sherman, *Rejection,* page 63 https://www.amazon.com/Rejection-James-R-Sherman-1982-04-30/dp/B01JXPC1SG

[18] Susan Ariel Rainbow Kennedy, *Succulent Wild Women, Dancing With Your Wonder-Full Self,* https://planetsark.com/

[19] Diego Perez, Twitter, https://twitter.com/YungPueblo/status/1118682962227290112, April 17, 2019

[20] World Health Organization (WHO), *https://www.who.int/about/who-we-are/frequently-asked-questions*

[21] Niklas Göke, Medium, https://medium.com/s/power-moves/you-dont-need-goals-you-need-a-theme-4a1a84de043b#:~:text=As%20Altucher%20sees%20it%2C%20your,the%20other%20from%20your%20results, 17 October, 2018

[22] Kelly Fryer, https://www.slideshare.net/KellyFryerBScMCIPDMA/change-your-mindset-in-6-steps, March 11, 2016

[23] Marcel, Schwantes, https://www.inc.com/marcel-schwantes/heres-tony-robbins-advice-on-how-to-dramatically-improve-your-communication-skills.html, June 14, 2019

[24] Tony Robbins, TonyRobbins.com, *Finding the Right Key,* https://www.tonyrobbins.com/leadership-impact/finding-the-right-key/

[25] Monika Walankiewicz, https://www.monikaw.com/blog/2017/10/24/lets-clear-the-confusion-habits-are-not-patterns, October 24, 2017

[26] Tony Robbins, *Are You Asking Yourself The Right Questions? How To Spark Catalytic Questions That Lead To Breakthrough Insights,* https://www.tonyrobbins.com/mind-meaning/are-you-asking-yourself-the-right-questions/

[27] Brené Brown, TED Talk, https://www.ted.com/talks/brene_brown_listening_to_shame/transcript?language=en, March 2012

[28] Arianna Huffington, https://thriveglobal.com/stories/microsteps-big-idea-too-small-to-fail-healthy-habits-willpower/, February 27, 2019

[29] David T. Neal, Wendy Wood, Jeffrey M. Quinn, https://dornsife.usc.edu/assets/sites/545/docs/Wendy_Wood_Research_Articles/Habits/Neal.Wood.Quinn.2006_Habits_a_repeat_performance.pdf, August 01, 2006

[30] Andrea Derler, PhD , Jennifer Ray, PhD, https://neuroleadership.com/your-brain-at-work/growth-mindset-deal-with-change, December 12, 2019

[31] Rick Hanson, https://www.rickhanson.net/find-your-north-star/

[32] Martha Beck, *Finding Your Own North Star, Claiming the Life You Were Meant to Love, Introduction, Page xiv*

[33] Martha Beck, *Finding Your Own North Star, Claiming the Life You Were Meant to Love, Introduction, Page xv*

[34] Jessica 'Chiara' Viscomi, M.A., Healthy Psych, *Your Own North Star: Finding Life Purpose and Passion,* https://healthypsych.com/your-own-north-star-finding-life-purpose-and-passion/, December 31, 2018

[35] Jessica 'Chiara' Viscomi, M.A., Healthy Psych, *Your Own North Star: Finding Life Purpose and Passion,* https://healthypsych.com/your-own-north-star-finding-life-purpose-and-passion/, December 31, 2018

[36] Kimberly Zapata, *How to Manifest Anything you Want or Desire,* https://www.oprahmag.com/life/a30244004/how-to-manifest-anything/, 22 December, 2020

[37] 1981, The Brothers Karamazov by Fyodor Dostoevsky, Translated by Andrew H. MacAndrew, Translation Copyright 1970, Book V: Pro and Contra, Chapter 5: The Grand Inquisitor, Quote Page 306 and 307, Bantam Books, New York.

[38] Harvard business Review, The President and the Board of Directors, Myles L. Mace https://hbr.org/1972/03/the-president-and-the-board-of-directors, March 1972

[39] Brené Brown, *Daring Greatly: How the Courage to Be Vulnerable Transforms the Way We Live, Love, Parent, and Lead,* 2012, page 36

[40] https://members.hustlecrew.co/brene-brown-on-the-power-of-vulnerability/

[41] Sylvester McNutt III, Instagram, https://www.instagram.com/p/CI0U-naL4ZM/, December 15, 2020

[42] University of Buffalo, School of Social Work, http://socialwork.buffalo.edu/resources/self-care-starter-kit/introduction-to-self-care.html

[43] Harvard Medical School, Harvard Health Publishing, https://www.health.harvard.edu/newsletter_article/direct-to-consumer-genetic-testing-kits, September 2010

[44] Amanda Macmillan, Time Magazine, https://time.com/5556071/gut-health-diet/, April 01, 2019

[45] National Center for Biotechnology Information, https://www.ncbi.nlm.nih.gov/pmc/articles/PMC6279019/, December 04, 2018

[46] Science Immunology, Vol. 5, Issue 45, eaay4209 https://immunology.sciencemag.org/content/5/45/eaay4209, Mar 06, 2020

[47] Esther Landhuis, Knowable Magazine, published on Scientific American, https://www.scientificamerican.com/article/gut-microbes-may-be-key-to-solving-food-allergies/, May 23, 2020

[48] Genova Diagnostics, *IGE Food Antibodies*, https://www.gdx.net/product/ige-food-allergy-test-blood

[49] The Cornucopia Institute, *Top 10 Most Common GMO Foods*, https://www.cornucopia.org/2013/06/top-10-most-common-gmo-foods/?gclid=CjOKCQiAnb79BRDgARIsAOVbhRopKX1SX7mgoqG0PusT1T2n-x2WzvLwh6F31ryAKLp_FiRdy76yEWQaArCuEALw_wcB, June 19, 2013.

[50] Food Allergy & Anaphylaxis Connection, https://www.foodallergyawareness.org/food-allergy-and-anaphylaxis/food-allergens/fish/#:~:text=Although%20any%20type%20of%20fish,reactions%20require%20urgent%20medical%20evaluation.

[51] Dr. Mark Hyman, M.D., Facebook, https://www.facebook.com/drmarkhyman/photos/a.163412217022869/3366570343373691/?type=3, May 30, 2020

[52] John Hopkins Medicine, *9 Benefits of Yoga*, https://www.hopkinsmedicine.org/health/wellness-and-prevention/9-benefits-of-yoga#:~:text=Yoga%20benefits%20heart%20health.,also%20be%20addressed%20through%20yoga.

[53] UC Davis Environmental Health Sciences Center, *What Environmental Factors Affect Health*, https://environmentalhealth.ucdavis.edu/communities/what-environmental-factors-affect-health

[54] EAT is an adapted summary of the Commission Food in The Anthropocene: the EAT-Lancet Commission on Healthy Diets From Sustainable Food Systems. The entire Commission can be found online at thelancet.com/commissions/EAT. https://eatforum.org/eat-lancet-commission/eat-lancet-commission-summary-report/

[55] Aaron E. Carroll, https://www.nytimes.com/2019/10/01/upshot/beef-health-climate-impact.html, October 01, 2019

[56] The Monday Campaigns, https://www.mondaycampaigns.org/meatless-monday/about

[57] Costello EK, Stagaman K, Dethlefsen L, Bohannan BJ, Relman DA. The application of ecological theory toward an understanding of the human microbiome. Science. 2012;336:1255–1262. [PMC free article] [PubMed] [Google Scholar]

[58] Dr. Tara Menon, M.D., The Ohio State University, Wexner Medical Center, https://wexnermedical.osu.edu/blog/everything-you-need-to-know-about-gut-health, August 07, 2020

59 Julia J. Tsuei, School of Public Health, John A. Burns School of Medicine, University of Hawaii, Kapiolani-Children's Medical Center, Honolulu, https://www.ncbi.nlm.nih.gov/pmc/articles/PMC1238216/, June 1978.

60 True Health Center for Functional Medicine, *What's the difference between Holistic, Naturopathic, Functional and Integrative Medicine?*, Kristine Burke, March 16, 2018. http://www.truehealthcfm.com/blog/whats-the-difference-between-holistic-naturopathic-functional-and-integrative-medicine,

61 Andrew Weil, M.D., DrWeil.com, https://www.drweil.com/health-wellness/balanced-living/meet-dr-weil/what-is-integrative-medicine/

62 The National Association of Nutrition Professionals, *What is Holistic Nutrition*, https://nanp.org/what-is-holistic-nutrition/

63 American College of Healthcare Sciences, *What is Holistic Nutrition?*, https://achs.edu/accredited-online-holistic-nutrition-degrees

64 EAT is an adapted summary of the Commission Food in The Anthropocene: the EAT-Lancet Commission on Healthy Diets From Sustainable Food Systems. The entire Commission can be found online at thelancet.com/commissions/EAT. https://eatforum.org/eat-lancet-commission/eat-lancet-commission-summary-report/

65 Katherine D. McManus, MS, RD, LDN, Harvard Medical School, Harvard Health Publishing, https://www.health.harvard.edu/blog/what-is-a-plant-based-diet-and-why-should-you-try-it-2018092614760, posted September 26, 2018, 10:30 AM, Updated August 31, 2020, 12:00 AM.

66 Fiona Lavelle, Michelle Spence, Lynsey Hollywood, Laura McGowan, Dawn Surgenor, Amanda McCloat, Elaine Mooney, Martin Caraher, Monique Raats, Moira Dean, *Learning cooking skills at different ages: a cross-sectional study*, https://pubmed.ncbi.nlm.nih.gov/27842556/

67 Hillary Clinton, Announcing Suspension of Presidential Campaign, https://www.americanrhetoric.com/speeches/hillaryclintoncampaignsuspensionspeech.htm, June 07, 2008

68 1992, A Return to Love: Reflections on the Principles of A Course in Miracles by Marianne Williamson, Chapter 7: Work, Quote Page 165, Published by HarperCollins, New York.

69 Steve Maraboli, Twitter, https://twitter.com/SteveMaraboli/status/931619951554777088/photo/1, November 17, 2017

70 Mark Mansson, MarkManson.net, https://markmanson.net/boundaries

71 Bock SA, Muñoz-Furlong A., Sampson H. Further fatalities caused by anaphylactic reactions to food, 2001- 2006. J Allergy Clin Immunol. 2007; 119(4): 1016-8. 2 Bock SA, Muñoz-Furlong A, Sampson HA. Fatalities due to anaphylactic reactions to foods. J Allergy Clin Immunol. 2001; 107(1): 191-3. 3 Sampson HA, Mendelson L, Rosen J. Fatal and

near-fatal anaphylactic reactions to food in children and adolescents. N Engl J Med.1992; 327(6): 380-4

[72] National Restaurant Association-commissioned survey by Product Evaluations, 2012 5 Lee YM, Xu H. Food allergy knowledge, attitudes, and preparedness among restaurants.

[73] Lee YM, Xu H. Food allergy knowledge, attitudes, and preparedness among restaurant managerial staff. J FoodServ Bus Res. 2015; 18(5): 454-469

[74] Food Allergy Research & Education, https://www.foodallergy.org/resources/food-allergies-and-restaurants

[75] Food Allergy and Intolerance Products – A Global Strategic Business Report. Global Industry Analysts, Inc., 2016.

[76] Food Allergy Research & Education, https://www.foodallergy.org/resources/food-allergies-and-restaurants

[77] Food Allergy Research & Education, https://www.foodallergy.org/resources/food-allergies-and-restaurants

[78] Food Safety News, *Mass Makes Restaurant Food Safety Priority,* https://www.foodsafetynews.com/2010/02/massachusetts-makes-restaurant-food-safety-high-priority/, 17 February, 2010

[79] FARE, Food Allergy Research & Education, https://www.foodallergy.org/resources/food-allergy-chef-cards

[80] Dhamma.org,*Vipassana Meditation,* https://www.dhamma.org/

[81] https://www.vridhamma.org/

[82] Food Allergy Research and Education, https://www.foodallergy.org/resources/facts-and-statistics, NIAID-Sponsored Expert Panel. Guidelines for the diagnosis and management of food allergy in the United States: Report of the NIAID-sponsored expert panel. J Allergy Clin Immunol. 2010; 126(6):S1- 58.

[83] W.S. Blatchley, *Boulder Reveries,* https://archive.org/details/boulderreveries00blatrich, page 70, 1906.

ABOUT THE AUTHOR

SONIA HUNT is a food allergy activist, TEDx speaker, tech marketing executive, and mentor to global organizations focused on social impact. She is the creator of the ***Three to Be™ program,*** a holistic health and well-being program that guides people with food allergies and food restrictions on how to **Be Healthy, Be Safe + Be Well™** (her mantra) to thrive in life. In her first book, *Nut Job: How I Crushed My Food Allergies To Thrive,* Sonia utilizes the *Three to Be™ program* to eliminate her food allergies holistically.

Sonia's life's work is at the intersection of humans, health, and technology, creating products and services that drive impact for people and the planet. Born and raised in Philadelphia, Pennsylvania, Sonia holds a Civil and Environmental Engineering degree from Drexel University. She is a fearless foodie and proud first-generation Indian-American who currently resides in San Francisco, California.

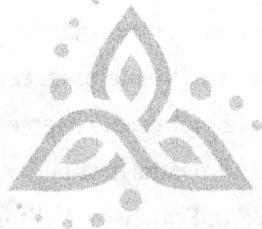

www.ingramcontent.com/pod-product-compliance
Lightning Source LLC
Chambersburg PA
CBHW030237030426
42336CB00009B/135